P9-DFH-341

Vitamins

Minerals

& Herbs

Reader's
Digest

Reader's Digest Association, Inc.
Pleasantville, New York / Montreal

Reader's Digest Project Staff

Senior Editor
Marianne Wait

Senior Designer
Judith Carmel

Production Technology Manager
Douglas A. Croll

Contributing Editor
Susan Carleton

Reader's Digest Health Publishing

Editorial Director
Christopher Cavanaugh

Art Director
Joan Mazzeo

Marketing Director
James H. Malloy

Vice President and General Manager
Shirrel Rhoades

The Reader's Digest Association, Inc.

Editor-in-Chief
Eric W. Schrier

President, North American Books and Home Entertainment
Thomas D. Gardner

Reader's Digest Book Produced by Rebus, Inc.

Publisher
Rodney Friedman

Senior Editor
Sandra Wilmot

Contributing Editor
Marya Dalrymple

Consulting Editors
Jeremy D. Birch, Andrea Peirce, Carol Weeg

Chief of Information Resources
Tom Damrauer

Production Database Manager
John Vasiliadis

Art Director
Timothy Jeffs

Art Associate
Bree Rock

Photographer
Lisa Koenig

Medical Board of Advisors

Chief Consultant
David Edelberg, M.D.

Consultants
Keith Berndtson, M.D., Roy R. Hall, M.D.,
Tony V. Lu, M.D., Mark Michaud, M.D.

Address any comments about Guide to Drugs and Supplements: Vitamins, Minerals, and Herbs to
Reader's Digest, Editorial Director, Reader's Digest Health Publishing
Reader's Digest Road
Pleasantville, NY 10570

To order additional copies of Guide to Drugs and Supplements: Vitamins, Minerals, and Herbs,
call 1-800-846-2100

Visit our website at www.rd.com

1 3 5 7 9 10 8 6 4 2

Copyrights © 2002 The Reader's Digest Association, Inc.
Copyrights © 2002 The Reader's Digest Association (Canada) Ltd.
Copyrights © 2002 Reader's Digest Association Far East Ltd.
Philippine Copyright 2002 Reader's Digest Association Far East Ltd.

All rights reserved. Unauthorized reproduction, in any manner,
is prohibited.

READER'S DIGEST and the Pegasus logo are registered trademarks of
The Reader's Digest Association, Inc.
Printed in the United States of America

Library of Congress Cataloging-in-Publication Data

Guide to drugs and supplements : vitamins, minerals, and herbs.
—Updated ed.
    p. cm.
Includes index.
ISBN 0-7621-0367-1
  1. Dietary supplements–Popular works. I. Title: Vitamins, minerals,
and herbs. II. Reader's Digest Association.

RM258.5 .G85 2002
615'.1–dc21

2001048892

Vitamins
Minerals
& Herbs

CONTENTS

▼

The editors, writers, medical consultants, and publisher have conscientiously and carefully tried to ensure that recommended measures and drug dosages in this book are accurate and conform to the standards that prevailed at the time of publication. The reader is advised, however, to consult with his or her doctors, pharmacists, and other health-care professionals, and to refer to any product information sheets that accompany his or her medications, be they prescription or over-the-counter. This advice should be taken with particular seriousness if the drug is a new one or one that is infrequently used. Because of the uniqueness of each patient, the need to take into account many clinical factors, and the continually evolving nature of drug information, use this book only as a general guide—along with the advice of your doctor, pharmacist, and other health-care professionals—to help make informed medical decisions.

THE NEW AGE OF NUTRITIONAL MEDICINES

▼

▼ THE CHANGING VIEW OF SUPPLEMENTS

The substances and products that we classify as supplements are by no means entirely new. Vitamins in pill form have been available for more than 50 years. Herbs, also known as botanicals or phytomedicines *(phyto* means "plant" in Latin), have been staples in the sickroom and the kitchen for centuries, and were the primary form of medicine in the United States until this century. Yet only a decade ago, most vitamin pills were fairly uniform "one-a-day" formulas, and herbal remedies often had to be concocted at home or purchased in out-of-the-way health-food stores.

◆ *Revived Interest*
Today, in the United States, "dietary supplements," as they are officially called, encompass a dizzying array of vitamins, minerals, and herbs, as well as other compounds that have been extracted or created from natural sources. (These compounds carry names such as glucosamine, coenzyme Q_{10}, and lycopene.)

Available without a prescription, supplements are sold in virtually every American supermarket and drugstore. Many malls and shopping areas have stores devoted entirely to supplements, and they can also be bought through catalogs and over the Internet. Annual supplement sales now exceed $16 billion and are expected to grow markedly in the future.

The public's intense interest in supplements is also apparent in the mass media. Newspapers, TV, and radio regularly highlight evidence of

their benefits—whether it is a review of 23 studies of St. John's wort for mild depression, a survey of the effects of ginkgo biloba on patients with dementia, or an article noting that the standard treatment for enlarged prostate in many European countries is not a conventional prescription drug, but the herb saw palmetto.

With all this attention and the rising sales of supplements, it isn't surprising that millions of Americans, including many doctors and scientists, have come to realize that substances such as garlic, echinacea, and grape seed extract, along with vitamins and minerals, are as beneficial to health as low-fat foods, exercise, and aspirin.

According to a number of surveys, one-third to one-half of all Americans now regularly use various forms of supplements as preventive medicine or as therapies for a wide range of ailments—from common complaints such as colds and headaches to more serious concerns, including arthritis, depression, and heart disease.

The fact that so many people are eager to try supplements, even when it is often hard to find reliable information, shows that major changes in health care have brought herbal and nutritional remedies closer to mainstream medicine. Traditionally, the medical community has been skeptical of these remedies and of alternative medicine. But that is changing.

◆ *Increased Research*
During the past decade, nutritional research has produced a flood of studies offering compelling evidence that specific foods and nutrients may help prevent, slow, or even reverse serious

diseases. For example, several large-scale studies from Harvard University have provided strong evidence that vitamin E supplementation is linked to lower rates of heart disease in men and women. From these results, experts have concluded that a higher level of vitamin E than is found in the average American diet (or can possibly be obtained from food alone) very likely offers some protection against heart disease.

These and similar studies cited throughout this book have changed the opinions of many scientists and other experts who were former skeptics. They now feel that supplementation with reasonable amounts of vitamins and minerals may increase a person's chances of staving off disease and enjoying optimal health.

◆ *Learning from Europe*
Though research into herbal remedies has lagged in the United States, in Europe herbs have been widely studied and scrutinized over the past 20 years, and standards have been established for their effectiveness and safety.

In Germany a special body of scientists and health professionals, known as Commission E, has been investigating the usefulness and safety of herbal remedies since 1978, gathering information from scientific literature, clinical trials, and medical associations. It has issued reports on some 300 herbs—and has found about two-thirds of them to be safe and effective.

This knowledge about the way herbs are used elsewhere has persuaded more American doctors and scientists to take a less dismissive view of herbal remedies.

◆ *Better Studies Still Needed*

Despite more extensive research, however, a number of benefits attributed to vitamins, minerals, and herbs remain unproved and controversial. Many doctors and researchers insist the studies on alternative remedies are not sufficiently rigorous. Furthermore, extreme claims of therapeutic benefits draw fire from critics—either because they are without merit or because they leave the impression that anything "natural" is harmless, which is not always the case. Many of the studies have been small in scale, and most don't offer a long-term evaluation of benefits and side effects.

On the other hand, as more studies are conducted, some impressive evidence is accumulating. In the research on the herb St. John's wort for mild to moderate depression, for example, 15 studies have compared an extract of the herb to a placebo, or neutral pill, in order to test for a placebo effect (an improvement in symptoms that some people experience because they believe they are receiving treatment, even though the pill is inactive).

In these studies, St. John's wort was found to be more effective than a placebo in treating relatively mild (although not severe) depressive symptoms. Other studies have shown that the herb works as well as standard prescription medications for treating mild depression. Moreover, side effects were infrequent and relatively innocuous—which is part of the appeal of many herbs.

◆ *Emphasis on Prevention*

Increasingly, there is a greater emphasis—backed by growing numbers of medical experts—on lifestyle choices as a critical factor in staying well. This has led more people to pay attention to diet, exercise, and weight control, which can help prevent or relieve common complaints, including backache and constipation. Many people have also quit smoking and limited their alcohol intake. All these changes can reduce the risk of serious ailments such as heart disease and cancer. (Researchers now think that three-quarters of all cancers result mainly from things people eat, drink, smoke, or encounter in the environment.)

Vitamins, minerals, and herbs can reinforce and enhance the benefit of these self-care measures, which are also essential for enjoying what might be termed optimal health—not simply the absence of illness, but the capacity to lead a full, vital, and productive life.

◆ *New Regulations*

In 1994 the United States government passed a new set of regulations called the Dietary Supplement Health and Education Act, which eased restrictions on the selling of vitamin, mineral, and herbal supplements. Reflecting and reinforcing the demands of consumers, the regulations have allowed supplement manufacturers to make certain claims about a product's health benefits without absolute proof of its therapeutic effects. The freedom to make these claims has been a key factor in the enormous number and variety of supplements that have come on the market.

▼ INTEGRATIVE HEALING

In recent years, Americans—including many consumers and some doctors—have become increasingly aware of the limitations of conventional medicine. Though medical science has found cures for many troubling health problems (including some infectious diseases that caused sickness and premature death on a grand scale), it has been less successful in combating chronic illnesses such as heart disease, cancer, and diabetes. And while drugs often offer potent treatments for many ailments, they also pose the risk of powerful and distressing side effects. In addition, medications can be very expensive, and the cost may be prohibitive for many patients.

 ### HEALTH PROFESSIONALS AND SUPPLEMENTS

Many doctors and nurses (as well as dietitians and other health professionals) who practice conventional medicine may act skeptical about alternative therapies. But as it turns out, many use vitamin and mineral supplements themselves.

In a survey of 181 cardiologists, nearly half of them were found to be regularly taking antioxidant vitamins. These included vitamins C and E, which have been linked to the prevention of heart disease and certain forms of cancer, as well as to control of a host of other ailments. A smaller percentage of the physicians (37%), however, recommended antioxidants routinely to their patients.

Another survey of 665 dietitians in Washington state found that nearly 60% took some nutritional supplement, either daily or occasionally.

◆ Beyond Managed Care

A good number of patients and doctors have also been frustrated by the growth of health maintenance organizations (HMOs) and similar managed-care health plans. Such plans have forced thousands of Americans, often against their will, to change doctors, and at the same time have restricted their choice. Doctors, in turn, chafe because their time with patients is limited. In fact, surveys show that more people are now complaining that their doctors don't pay enough attention to them. Furthermore, many managed-care plans don't provide the same level of coverage that traditional insurers once did, so patients frequently have to pay more out of their own pockets for services rendered.

As awareness of these shortcomings has grown, consumers have become more enthusiastic about alternative approaches to treating ailments. Generally these methods—which include therapies such as chiropractic, acupuncture, and massage, as well as supplements—are considered less invasive and more "holistic" (treating the whole person, rather than simply suppressing symptoms) than conventional treatments. As you read this book, you will see that supplements often act to enhance the body's own defenses. An herb you take to help treat an infection, for example, often doesn't directly kill bacteria (as an antibiotic would), but rather strengthens your immune system so your body can kill the bacteria.

Alternative therapies are also typically less expensive than conventional treatments; supplements, in particular, usually cost far less than prescription drugs, and may even be cheaper than some over-the-counter medications. Alternative therapies, such as acupuncture and chiropractic, are now covered by some health-care plans.

Behind many of these alternative choices in healing is a common perspective: The body has amazing powers of self-repair. According to this view, supplements, when used wisely, can bolster the body's immune system to prevent disease. If a health problem does occur, they can also enhance and accelerate self-healing.

◆ Doctors Reassess

Consumers have shown that they want to try alternative approaches, and physicians are slowly responding to demands from patients. However, rather than thinking of supplements and other less-established remedies as "alternatives" that exclude conventional treatments, some doctors are attempting to integrate the two, so that alternative medicine options can work hand-in-hand with Western medicine. (Recognizing this development, the federal government in 1992 established an Office of Alternative Medicine, which funds serious research at major medical centers to study complementary, and alternative, treatments for a variety of ailments.)

In an integrative approach, ideally, you and your doctor work together to reach a decision about which supplement or other therapy to use for treating your particular health problem (see the box opposite). On the other hand, many doctors and other members of the medical establishment are still resistant to complementary healing methods. Thus, there is no single reliable entity to supply advice about these remedies. In the end, it is up to consumers to acquaint themselves with the various types of complementary therapies, including supplements, that are now available.

▼ SUPPLEMENTS—OR DRUGS?

One reflection of the mainstream popularity of herbal and nutritional supplements is that not only do most drugstores in the United States stock them, these products are often shelved right next to over-the-counter drugs. Both types of products make health-related claims, and both are supplied in forms such as capsules, tablets, or powders. So a consumer may well ask, what's the difference?

◆ No Simple Answer

Concerned about the marketing of supplements, legislators have made a concerted effort to distinguish them from pharmaceutical drugs. By law, manufacturers of drugs (both over-the-counter and prescription) can make explicit claims about a product's ability to prevent or treat a recognized medical condition—for example, alleviating headaches or relieving heartburn. But such claims can be made only after a lengthy approval process by the Food and Drug Administration (FDA), which verifies the drug's safety and effectiveness.

According to the Dietary Supplement Health and Education Act, which regulates the marketing of such products, supplements are intended to "supplement the diet" and must contain one or more of the following: vitamins, minerals, herbs (also called botanicals), amino acids, and/or other nutritional substances. Supplements are not subjected to the rigorous testing and scrutiny that drugs receive, and therefore the labels on supplements cannot promise to cure or prevent diseases. However the labels *can* list potential benefits that affect bodily functions, such as "promoting healthy cholesterol" or "aiding digestion."

YOU AND YOUR DOCTOR: SOME GUIDELINES

A growing number of doctors and patients are embracing an integrative, or complementary, approach to treating health problems. This entails carefully weighing both conventional and alternative methods in order to create a strategy best suited to a patient's particular needs.

For example, a person with high blood pressure finds that the side effects from a prescription drug are distressing, so he and his doctor decide on a course of therapy that combines supplements with other lifestyle adjustments to see if it can effectively lower the blood pressure with less distress.

Traditionally medical schools teach their students very little about nutritional and herbal therapies. But because professional journals and postgraduate courses for physicians are giving these forms of treatment increasing attention, many doctors are becoming better acquainted with them.

Be sure to keep the following guidelines in mind when considering various treatment options and working with your doctor:

• **Don't diagnose yourself.** If you have symptoms that suggest an illness, see a doctor—either an M.D., a D.O. (doctor of osteopathic medicine), or a trained and licensed doctor of naturopathy.

• **Talk to your doctor.** Be sure to report all of your symptoms; never hide anything from your doctor. Also, be sure to tell your doctor about any supplements that you are now taking, because some of them might not interact well with conventional drugs that you may be asked to try. Even if your doctor isn't receptive to nutritional remedies, you should still discuss any supplements you are already taking or thinking of using, particularly if you have a chronic condition such as asthma, diabetes, migraine, heart disease, or high blood pressure.

• **Don't stop treatment.** Some supplements may complement, or even replace, conventional drugs. But you should never discontinue or alter the dosage of any prescribed medication without first consulting your doctor.

• **Recognize when conventional methods are best.** It can be foolish—and sometimes even dangerous—to seek alternative options for medical conditions that Western-trained doctors excel in treating or preventing. These include medical and surgical emergencies, physical injuries, acute infections, sexually transmitted diseases, kidney infections, reconstructive surgery, and serious illnesses, such as polio and diphtheria, that can be prevented with immunizations.

Of course, such statements (which are called "structure-function claims") usually imply treatment for a particular health problem. People who are worried about high cholesterol levels and heart disease, for example, are more likely to respond to anything promoting "healthy" cholesterol. Such links are frequently spelled out in manufacturers' brochures and in supplement sales materials, as well as in news reports and various publications.

◆ *Truthfulness of Claims*

Whether the assertions on supplement labels are always true is an issue that regulators have wrestled with but not resolved. The law states that all claims must be "truthful and not misleading,"

and in many cases, there is some scientific basis for such claims. But supplement manufacturers don't have to submit any data in advance of making a claim; they merely need to have the evidence on hand. Hence, labels must contain a statement that the claims " . . . have not been evaluated by the Food and Drug Administration."

So, if many supplements do, in fact, act like drugs and are often used as drugs, why aren't they tested and marketed as drugs? It's because vitamins, minerals, herbs, and other supplements can be derived directly from plants and other natural sources—and therefore can't be patented. Thus there is little financial incentive for drug or supplement makers to spend

millions on the research and approval process required for a nutrient to obtain the status of a drug. Once an herb or herb component receives FDA approval, any company can then sell the same product.

Government regulation of supplements will no doubt evolve as their use continues to grow and as more is learned about their effects. At some point, American regulations and practices may move closer to those of a number of European countries, where herbal remedies are examined and formulated with more rigor. For now, it is helpful to remember that the claims made on most supplement labels are not equivalent to—or as stringent as—those on most drug labels.

▼ PLENTY OF GOOD REASONS

Many people take a multivitamin supplement as nutritional "insurance" against deficiencies. But recent research provides additional reasons for using a variety of supplements, including herbs, and indicates that optimal levels may be higher than conventional wisdom has long dictated.

If you're basically healthy, should you take supplements on a regular basis? And if you develop an ailment, can you really expect supplements to help? What follows is a summary of the major benefits most people can expect from using the supplements covered in this book.

▼ ENHANCING YOUR DIET

Conventional wisdom holds that as long as people who are healthy eat well enough to avoid specific nutri-tional deficiencies, they don't need to supplement their diet. The only thing they have to do is consume foods that meet the RDAs—Recommended Dietary Allowances—and other guidelines for vitamin and mineral intakes developed by the federal government (see the box on page 13).

But even if one accepts the government's standards for vitamin and mineral intake as adequate for good health, the evidence is overwhelming that most people don't come close to meeting those nutritional requirements. Surveys show that only 9% of Americans eat five daily servings of fresh fruits and vegetables—the amount recommended for obtaining the minimum level of nutrients believed necessary to prevent illness.

Average calcium consumption in the United States and Canada is estimated to be about 60% of the current suggested level of 1,000 mg for adults ages 19 to 50—and far below the 1,200 mg recommended for men and women ages 51 to 70 and older.

According to a review of national data by experts at the University of California, Berkeley, people often make food choices that are nutritionally poor: For example, they are more likely to select french fries than broccoli as a vegetable and will typically opt for a soft drink over a glass of skim milk as a beverage. Not only can these and other foods contribute too much fat and sugar to the diet, but they can also result in less than optimal intakes of vitamins, minerals, and disease-fighting phytochemicals. The diets of many Americans, these experts note, contain just half the recommended amounts of magnesium and folic acid. Vitamins A, C, and B_6, as well as iron and zinc, are other nutrients that surveys show are at low levels in the American diet.

ANTIOXIDANTS: POWERFUL FREE-RADICAL FIGHTERS

Although oxygen is essential for life, it can also have adverse effects on your body. In the normal process of using oxygen, chemical changes occur in the body that create reactive unstable oxygen molecules called free radicals; these can damage cells and structures within cells, including genetic material (DNA).

Free radicals also may form in response to external factors (cigarette smoke and alcohol), pollutants (nitrogen oxide and ozone), and ultraviolet light and other forms of radiation (including X rays). If the genetic material in cells is affected, it can be replicated in new cells, contributing to cancer and other serious health problems. Free radicals may also weaken artery walls, allowing fatty deposits that can lead to heart disease to collect.

Cells have special agents for combating free radicals and repairing molecular damage. These are called antioxidants. A good deal of recent research suggests that antioxidants may play important roles in preventing or delaying heart disease, cancer, and other ills and may even slow the effects of aging.

Vitamins C and E are perhaps the best-known antioxidants. The mineral selenium is also an antioxidant, as are carotenoids such as beta-carotene and lycopene. Enzymes and certain other compounds (such as glutathione) manufactured by the cells themselves also act as antioxidants. A number of other substances, including certain herbs, may act as antioxidants as well. For example, green tea, grape seed extract, and ginkgo biloba (among others) are all thought to have antioxidant properties.

◆ Filling Nutritional Gaps

Even with the best nutritional planning, it is difficult to maintain a diet that meets the RDAs for all nutrients. For example, vegetarians, who as a group are healthier than meat eaters (and who tend to avoid junk foods lacking in vitamins and minerals), still may be deficient in some nutrients, such as iron, calcium, and vitamin B_{12}. And most people who want to maintain a healthy low-fat diet will have a problem obtaining the recommended amounts of vitamin E from their food alone, because so many of the food sources for vitamin E are high in fat.

Another complication is that a balanced diet may not contain the more specialized substances—fish oils, soy isoflavones, or alpha-lipoic acid—that researchers think may promote health. For generally healthy people who can't eat a well-balanced diet every day, a supplement can fill in these nutritional gaps or boost the nutrients they consume from adequate to optimal.

There are various other reasons why people who maintain good eating habits might benefit from a daily supplement. Some experts now believe that exposure to environmental pollutants—from car emissions to industrial chemicals and wastes—can cause damage in myriad ways inside the body at the cellular level, destroying tissues and depleting the body of nutrients. Many supplements, particularly those that act as antioxidants, can help control the cell and tissue damage that follows toxic exposure (see the box opposite). Recent evidence also indicates that certain medications, excess alcohol, smoking, and persistent stress may interfere with the absorption of certain key nutrients. And even an excellent diet would be unable to make up for such a shortfall.

TOO MANY BENEFITS: **TOO GOOD TO BE TRUE?**

When you see a supplement label that lists a variety of functions and benefits for a single herb or substance, you might wonder if this is more marketing hype than facts. You can't rely entirely on label claims, because they aren't scrutinized for accuracy by the government or any other agency. But as you will see in reading this book, some supplements do have multiple effects that are well documented.

Consider an herb such as green tea. According to many studies, its benefits may include helping control several cancers, including colon and pancreatic cancer; protecting against heart disease; inhibiting the action of bacteria; and acting as an antioxidant to bolster the immune system. All of these benefits aren't too surprising, given that researchers have identified various active components in green tea.

You should be aware that many common medications were initially developed for one purpose. As more people take the drugs and their effects are studied, new uses come to light. Imagine a drug that can cure headaches, relieve arthritis, help prevent heart disease, ease the pain of athletic injuries, and reduce the risk of colon cancer. It's aspirin, of course—and its precursor came from an herbal source, the bark of the white willow tree.

▼ PREVENTING DISEASE AND SLOWING AGING

For many years, it was thought that a lack of nutrients was linked only to specific deficiency diseases such as scurvy, a condition marked by soft gums and loose teeth that is caused by too little vitamin C. In the past three decades, however, thousands of scientific studies have indicated that specific nutrients appear to play key roles in the prevention of a number of chronic ailments common in contemporary Western societies.

Many recent studies highlighting the disease-fighting potential of different nutrients are mentioned in this book. What most of these studies reveal is that the level of nutrients associated with disease prevention is often significantly higher than the current RDIs or RDAs. To achieve these higher levels, the participants in these studies often had to depend on using supplements.

◆ The Role of Antioxidants

In slowing or preventing the development of disease, some experts suggest that nutrients, particularly the antioxidants, can also delay the wear and tear of aging by reducing the damage done to cells. This idea does not mean vitamin E or coenzyme Q_{10}, for example, are "youth potions." But several recent studies, including work done at the Nutritional Immunological Laboratory at Tufts University, have found that supplementation with single nutrients, such as vitamin E, or with multivitamin and mineral formulas, appear to improve immune response among older people.

For example, the results of a study of 11,178 elderly subjects, conducted by researchers at the National Institute on Aging, showed that the use of vitamin E was associated with a lowered risk of total mortality, and especially of death from heart disease. In fact, vitamin E users were only half as likely to die of heart disease as those taking no supplements. In addition, there is evidence that antioxidant supplements are effective in lowering the risk of cataracts and macular degeneration, two age-related vision conditions.

Other supplements that serve as high-potency antioxidants against aging disorders include the mineral selenium, carotenoids, flavonoids, certain amino acids, and coenzyme Q_{10}. Some experts also believe that the herb ginkgo biloba may improve many age-related symptoms, especially those involving reduced blood flow, such as dizziness, impotence, and short-term memory loss. Substances found in echinacea and other herbs are reported to strengthen the immune system, and phytoestrogens such as soy isoflavones are thought to help delay or forestall some of the effects of menopause, as well as to help prevent cancer and heart disease.

▼ TREATING AILMENTS

Practitioners of complementary medicine often recommend supplements for a wide range of health problems affecting virtually every body system. For most of these conditions, conventional physicians would be more likely to prescribe drugs. Some disorders, however, routinely require supplements. For example, iron may be prescribed for some types of anemia, vitamin A (in the drug isotretinoin, or Accutane) for severe acne, and high doses of the B vitamin niacin for reducing high cholesterol levels.

In this book, certain vitamins and minerals are suggested for the treatment of specific ailments. However, the use of supplements as remedies, especially for serious conditions, is controversial. Most doctors practicing conventional medicine are skeptical of supplements' efficacy and believe it is sometimes dangerous to rely on them. But based on published data and their clinical observations, nutritionally oriented physicians and practitioners think the use of these supplements is justified—and that to wait years for unequivocal proof to appear would be wasting valuable time. Even so, until there is more consistent evidence available, you should be careful about depending on nutritional supplements alone to treat any serious ailment.

◆ Age-Old Remedies
Despite these cautions, it is important to note that for thousands of years, various cultures have employed herbs for soothing, relieving, or even curing many common health problems, a fact not ignored by medical science. The pharmaceutical industry, after all, arose as a consequence of people using herbs as medicine. Recent studies suggest that a number of the claims made for herbs have validity, and the pharmacological actions of the herbs covered in this book are often well documented by clinical studies as well as historical practice. In Europe, a number of herbal remedies, including St. John's wort, ginkgo biloba, and saw palmetto, now are accepted and prescribed as medications for treating disorders such as allergies, depression, impotence, and even heart disease. Of course, even herbs and other supplements with proven therapeutic effects should be used judiciously (see the safety guidelines box on page 19).

▼ WHAT SUPPLEMENTS WON'T DO

Despite the many promising benefits that supplements offer, it's important to note their limits—and to question some of the extravagant claims currently being made for them.

◆ Not Food Stand-ins
As the word itself suggests, supplements are not meant to replace the nutrients available from foods. They can't counteract a high intake of saturated fat (which has been linked to an increased risk of heart disease and cancer), and they can't replace nutrients found in foods you ignore. Also, although scientists have extracted a number of disease-fighting phytochemical compounds from fruits, vegetables, and other foods, there may be many others that are yet undiscovered—ones you can get only from foods. In addition, some of the known compounds may work only in combination with others in various foods, rather than as single isolated ingredients in supplement form.

◆ Not Magic Lifestyle Bullets
Supplements won't compensate for habits known to contribute to ill health, such as smoking or a lack of exercise. Optimal health requires a wholesome lifestyle—particularly if, as people get older, they are intent on aging well.

◆ Not Weight-Loss Miracles
Weight-loss preparations may be popular, but it's questionable whether any of them can help you shed pounds without the right food choices and regular exercise. Products that claim to "burn fat" won't burn enough on their own for significant weight loss.

◆ *Not Performance Boosters*

Similarly, claims of improving performance, whether physical or mental, are very difficult to back up—and any "enhancement" will be a limited one at best in a healthy person. Though a supplement may boost mental functioning in someone experiencing mild to severe memory loss, it may have a negligible effect on the memory or concentration of most adults. Likewise, a supplement that combats fatigue isn't going to turn the average jogger into an endurance athlete. Nor is it clear that "aphrodisiac" supplements favored by many men today are effective for enhancing sexual performance if you aren't suffering from some form of sexual dysfunction.

◆ *Not Cure-Alls*

To date, no supplements have been found to cure any serious diseases—including cancer, heart disease, high blood pressure, diabetes, or AIDS. The right supplement, however, may help to improve a chronic condition, such as migraine or osteoarthritis, and it may also help to relieve symptoms such as pain or inflammation. Supplements are also good for treating minor wounds and burns.

The important thing to remember is that before using supplements for any ailment you first need to consult a health professional for treatment.

RDAs, DVs, RDIs, AIs: **WHAT DO THOSE NUMBERS MEAN?**

Over the years, government-sponsored committees of nutritional experts, including those in the National Academy of Sciences and the Food and Drug Administration, have established various guidelines for the amounts of vitamins and minerals needed by most individuals to achieve and maintain good health. Understanding what these different standards signify can be confusing. All of them, however, represent similar values based on the "gold standard" of vitamin and mineral intake: the RDAs, or Recommended Dietary Allowances.

Early standards

The first RDAs were developed in 1941 and have been revised periodically by the Food and Nutrition Board of the National Research Council. The RDAs are different for men, women, and children, for different age groups, and for pregnant or lactating women. Some years ago, a new standard, the Reference Daily Intake, or RDI, was created for each nutrient. The RDIs are intended to represent nutrient needs of an average healthy person. In most cases they are the highest levels of adult RDAs, though they also take into account other guidelines.

On many labels of vitamin and mineral supplements (as well as on food labels), you will see a set of figures under the heading "% Daily Value," or DV. The Daily Value is simply a percentage of the RDI. It tells you how much of a particular nutrient is supplied by a dose of the supplement (or, in the case of food labels, by a serving of food). The sample label on page 17 shows how the DV typically appears.

The RDIs replace an older value called the U.S. RDA. Though this value is no longer used for foods, some supplement labels continue to state nutrient values as a percentage of the U.S. RDA.

Slightly revised guidelines

Recently, the Food and Nutrition Board introduced a new set of values called Dietary Reference Intakes (DRIs). These include RDAs as well as Adequate Intakes (AIs) for certain nutrients for which there is not enough evidence to establish an RDA. In releasing new recommendations, the board raised some RDA levels to take into account the prevention of disorders other than deficiency diseases. For example, the latest recommendation for folic acid for women age 18 and older has been raised from 180 mcg to 400 mcg—a level thought to protect against certain birth defects and heart disease.

In each of the vitamin and mineral profiles (under "How Much You Need"), you'll find the RDA or Adequate Intake for that nutrient. Deficiencies from getting too little, and any adverse effects from getting too much, are also indicated, when known.

Are they enough?

Remember that the RDAs, RDIs, and DRIs are recommendations, not requirements, for large groups of people. The values are at a level assumed to supply the nutrient needs of most people, plus a generous margin of safety. Many experts, however, think RDAs (especially those for vitamins) are still far too low for maintaining optimal health or for treating certain diseases. Also, the values don't take into account such variables as smoking, alcohol consumption, exposure to pollutants, and medication use, which can interfere with nutrient absorption.

▼ TYPES OF SUPPLEMENTS

Anyone who has strolled down a dietary supplement aisle is aware of—and possibly overwhelmed by—the huge variety of products available. Counting different brands and combinations of supplements, there are now literally thousands of choices. Though you'll hardly encounter this many products in any one location, even the relatively limited selection in your local supermarket can be very confusing.

One reason for so much variety is that marketers are constantly trying to make their own brands stand out, so they devise different dosages, new combinations of ingredients, and creatively worded claims for their products. At the same time, scientists have found new and better ways of extracting nutritional components from plants and synthesizing nutrients in a laboratory—discoveries that have resulted in many new products.

To make informed decisions, it's essential to understand the terms used on supplement labels (see the box on page 17), as well as the properties and characteristics of specific supplements, which you will find in the individual supplement profiles (beginning on page 22). But to avoid feeling overwhelmed by all the choices facing you, it's first useful to learn about the basic types of supplements that are available and the key functions they perform in helping to keep you healthy.

◆ Vitamins
Vitamins are chemically organic substances (meaning they contain carbon) essential for regulating both the metabolic functions within the cells and the biochemical processes that release energy from food. In addition, evidence is accumulating that certain vitamins also act as antioxidants—substances that protect tissues from cell damage and possibly help prevent a number of degenerative diseases (see pages 10 to 12).

With a few exceptions (notably vitamins D and K), the body cannot manufacture vitamins on its own, so they must be ingested in food or nutritional supplements. There are 13 known vitamins that can be categorized as either fat-soluble (A, D, E, and K) or water-soluble (eight B vitamins and vitamin C). The distinction is important because the body stores fat-soluble vitamins for relatively long periods (months or even years); on the other hand, water-soluble vitamins (except for vitamin B_{12}) remain in the body for a short period of time and must be replenished more frequently.

◆ Minerals
Minerals are present in your body in small amounts: All together, they add up to only 4% of body weight. Yet these inorganic substances, which are found in the earth's crust as well as in many foods, are essential for a wide range of vital processes, from basic bone formation to the normal functioning of the heart and digestive system. A number of minerals have also been linked to the prevention of cancer, osteoporosis, and other chronic illnesses.

Just as with vitamins, people must replenish their mineral supply either through foods or through supplements. The body contains over 60 different minerals, but only 22 are thought to be essential. Of these, seven—including calcium, chloride, magnesium, phosphorus, potassium, sodium, and sulfur—are usually designated macrominerals, or major minerals. The other 15 minerals are termed trace minerals, or microminerals, because the amount that the body requires each day for good health is extremely tiny (usually it's measured in micrograms, or millionths of a gram).

◆ Herbs
Herbal supplements are prepared from plants—often using the leaves, stems, roots, and/or bark, as well as the buds and flowers. Known for centuries as medicinal agents, many plant parts can be used in their natural form, or they can be refined into tablets, capsules, powders, liquids, and other supplement formulations.

Many herbs have several active compounds that interact with one another to produce a therapeutic effect. An herbal supplement may contain all of the compounds found in a plant, or just one or two of the isolated compounds that have been successfully extracted. For some herbs, however, the active agents simply haven't been identified, so using the complete herb is necessary to obtain all its benefits.

Of the hundreds of remedies that are surfacing in the current rebirth of herbal medicines, the majority are being used to treat chronic or mild health problems. Increasingly, herbs are also being employed to attain or maintain good health—for example, to enhance the immune system, to help maintain low blood cholesterol levels, or to safeguard against fatigue. Less commonly, some herbs are now recommended as complementary therapy for acute or severe diseases.

◆ *Nutritional Supplements*

These nutrients include a diverse group of supplement products. Some, such as fish oils, are food substances that scientists have concluded possess disease-fighting potential. Flavonoids, soy isoflavones, and carotenoids are phytochemicals—compounds found in fruits and vegetables that work to lower the risk of disease and that may, in addition, alleviate symptoms of some ailments, such as heart disease and menopausal problems.

Other nutritional supplements, such as DHEA, melatonin, and coenzyme Q_{10}, are substances present in the body that can be re-created synthetically in a laboratory. A similar example is acidophilus, a "friendly" bacterium in the body that, taken as a supplement, may aid in the treatment of digestive disorders. Amino acids, which are building blocks for proteins and may play a role in strengthening the immune system and in promoting health in other ways, have been known to scientists for many years. Only fairly recently, however, have they been marketed as individual dietary supplements.

The many choices available today allow you to find supplements that are safe, effective, and convenient. Some of these "special" formulations, however, appear to provide little additional benefit, and they are frequently not worth the extra expense.

Supplements come in a variety of forms that affect both their ease of use and, in some cases, their rate of absorption by the body. (Each supplement profile lists the available forms for that supplement.)

▼ COMMON FORMS

In general, tablets and capsules are the most convenient forms of vitamin, mineral, or nutritional supplements to take, but there are other options as well. You can also purchase whole herbs and make up your own formulations. Most of the prepackaged forms described here are readily available in drugstores, supermarkets, and health-food stores. Whole herbs can be purchased at herb stores and some health-food stores.

Tablets and Capsules Stored away from heat and light, tablets and capsules will generally keep longer than other supplement forms. It's important to be aware that vitamin tablets often contain generally inert additives known as excipients, in addition to the vitamin itself. These compounds bind, preserve, or give bulk to the supplement, and help the tablets break down more quickly in your stomach. Increasingly, supplements are also available in capsule-shaped, easy-to-swallow tablets called "caplets."

The fat-soluble vitamins A, D, and E are typically packaged in "softgel" capsules. Other vitamins and minerals are processed into powders or liquids and then encapsulated. Like tablets, capsules are easy to use and store. They also tend to have fewer additives than

ABOUT **THE LABEL CLAIMS**

Advertising claims imply that vitamins derived from "natural" sources (such as vitamin E from soybeans) are better than "synthetic" vitamins created chemically in a laboratory. They may state that their natural products are more potent or more efficiently absorbed—and manufacturers generally charge more for natural products. But what is "natural"?

Actually, most supplements, no matter what their source, undergo processing with chemicals in laboratories. Some products labeled "natural" are really synthetic vitamins with plant extracts or minute amounts of naturally derived vitamins mixed in. Hence, "vitamin C from rose hips" may be mostly synthetic. And even the most natural products must be refined and processed, so they contain some additives. In any case, there's no difference chemically between natural and synthetic vitamins—nor can your body distinguish between the two.

Some researchers consider natural sources of vitamin E more effective than synthetic versions. But the International Units (IUs) used to measure vitamin E's potency take this into account, so a capsule designated to provide 400 IUs will have that potency no matter what its source.

Generally, there's no reason to pay more for supplements advertised as "natural." The cheapest synthetic vitamin or mineral supplement will give you the same benefit. Of course, the cheapest supplement isn't always the best. You should check the excipients, or additives, in a supplement to be sure that you aren't allergic to any—and you may have to pay more for a supplement with fewer of these inert filler ingredients.

tablets, and there is some evidence that they dissolve more readily (though this doesn't mean they are better absorbed by the body—just that they may be absorbed more quickly).

If you are taking herbs, you can avoid the taste of the herb (which some people don't like) if you use tablets or capsules. Herbal tablets and capsules are both prepared using either a whole herb or an extract of the herb containing a high concentration of the herb's active components. In either of these forms, the constituents are ground into a powder that can then be pressed into tablets or encapsulated.

Some herbs come in enteric-coated capsules, which pass through the stomach to the small intestine before dissolving. This minimizes potential gastrointestinal discomfort and, for some herbs, enhances their absorption into the bloodstream.

Sublingual Tablets A few supplements, such as vitamin B_{12}, are formulated to dissolve under the tongue. This process provides quick absorption into the bloodstream without interference from stomach acids and digestive enzymes.

Powders People who find pills hard to swallow can use powders, which can be mixed into juice or water, or stirred into food and taken with meals. (Ground seeds such as psyllium and flaxseed often come in powdered form.) Powders also allow dosages to be adjusted easily. Because they may have fewer binders or additives than tablets or capsules, powders are useful for those individuals who are allergic to certain substances. In addition, powders are often cheaper than tablets or capsules.

Tinctures and Liquid Extracts Tinctures are made by soaking the whole herb or parts of it in water and ethyl alcohol. The alcohol extracts and concentrates the herb's active components. (Nonalcoholic concentrations can be made using glycerin.)

Liquid extracts are more concentrated than tinctures. Again, the herb is soaked in a solvent such as water and alcohol, but then the alcohol is distilled away, usually by a vacuum process that doesn't heat the herb and change its potency.

Chewables Such supplements (usually packaged as flavored wafers) are particularly recommended for those who have trouble getting pills down. In this book, the most common wafer form is DGL, a licorice preparation. DGL is activated by saliva, so the wafers must be chewed, not simply swallowed.

Lozenges A number of supplements are available as lozenges or drops. These are intended to dissolve gradually in the mouth, either for ease of use or, in the case of zinc lozenges, to help in the treatment of colds and flu.

Oils Oils extracted from herbs can be commercially distilled to form potent concentrations for external use. These so-called essential oils are placed in a neutral "carrier" oil, such as almond oil, before use on the skin. Essential herbal oils should never be ingested. The exception is peppermint oil. A few drops on the tongue are recommended for bad breath, and capsules can be beneficial for irritable colon.

Gels, Ointments, and Creams Gels and ointments, made from fats or oils of aromatic herbs, can be applied to the skin to soothe rashes, heal bruises or wounds, and serve other therapeutic purposes. Creams are light mixtures of oil and water that are partially absorbed by the skin, allowing it to breathe while keeping in moisture. Creams can be used for moisturizing dry skin, for cleansing, and for relieving rashes, insect bites, or sunburn.

Tea Infusions and Decoctions Less concentrated than liquid forms, herbal tea infusions are brewed from the softer parts of the herb—the fresh or dried flowers, or the stems or leaves; these can be purchased in bulk or in tea bags. Be sure to use very hot (not boiling) water when preparing a tea infusion to preserve the beneficial oils that can be dissipated by the steam of boiling water. Also let the tea sit covered for 5 to 10 minutes. Decoctions, which use the tougher parts of an herb (roots, twigs, or bark), are simmered for at least half an hour.

For maximum potency drink herbal teas soon after brewing them, or store them in tightly sealed glass jars in the refrigerator for up to three days.

◆ *Special Formulations*
You will usually pay more for a supplement if the label says "timed-release" or "chelated." Does it provide extra benefits? Not often, according to available data. If you do decide to purchase one of these products keep the following information in mind:

Timed-Release Formulas These formulas contain microcapsules that gradually break down to release the vitamin steadily into the bloodstream over roughly 2 to 10 hours, depending on the product. ("Sustained-release" describes the same process.)

There are no reliable studies showing that timed-release formulas are

HOW TO READ **A SUPPLEMENT LABEL**

It wasn't that long ago that labels on dietary supplements provided scant information and made unsubstantiated claims. Recent rulings by the Food and Drug Administration (FDA), however, have changed all that.

All supplement labels now are required to carry a "Supplements Facts" box listing ingredients by weight. For those nutrients with an established Reference Daily Intake (RDI), the percentage must be listed and expressed as Percent Daily Value (DV). In the case of plant (or herbal) medicines, the label must identify the part used.

In addition, a number of other requirements must be followed. The information accompanying the label at right explains some of the key FDA rulings.

It is important to note that the FDA requirements are aimed at providing consumers with more reliable and consistent information about the tens of thousands of products designed to "supplement" the diet, such as vitamins, minerals, herbs, and amino acids.

The new labeling requirements do not, however, mean that supplements must withstand strict government scrutiny as prescription and over-the-counter drugs do. Supplement manufacturers are expected to ensure that their preparations are safe, but most products need not undergo an elaborate testing and review process. The government can step in only if a supplement appears to pose a health risk or makes drug-like claims for treating disease.

The bottom line: Stick with products made by reputable manufacturers that you trust. Never use products with labels that do not give you enough information for careful use.

HIGH POTENCY FORMULA FOR WOMEN

Antioxidant dietary supplement

STRENGTHENS CELLS, SUPPORTS BONE HEALTH, PROTECTS AGAINST OXIDATIVE DAMAGE*

*This statement has not been evaluated by the Food and Drug Administration. This product is not intended to diagnose, treat, cure, or prevent any disease.

Antioxidant vitamins C and E

100 tablets

DIRECTIONS: Take two (2) tablets daily

Supplement Facts

Serving Size: 2 tablets

Amount Per Tablet		% Daily Value
VITAMIN A	5000 I.U.	100%
VITAMIN C	250 mg	417%
VITAMIN E	200 I.U.	667%
CALCIUM	250 mg	25%
FRESH BLACK COHOSH EXTRACT (4:1 extract in 70% ethanol)	40 mg	*

* Daily Value not established

INGREDIENTS: ascorbic acid, d-alpha tocopheryl acetate, sodium selenate.

STORAGE: Keep tightly closed in dry place.

KEEP OUT OF REACH OF CHILDREN

EXPIRATION DATE: 11/02

Manufacturer or distributor's name, address, and zip code

A high potency label can be added to a product, such as this antioxidant formula, if at least two-thirds of the nutrients meet the Daily Value—and those nutrients must be identified. A single-nutrient product must contain 100% or more of the nutrients that meet the Daily Value. Most vitamin and mineral supplements easily meet this standard. For herbs, no Daily Value has been established.

Structure-function claims can describe only a product's effects on the body's structure or function, and not its potential health benefits.

A standard FDA disclaimer must accompany the vague and often meaningless structure-function claims that are allowed.

The Supplement Facts box, similar to the Nutrition Facts box on foods, lists key ingredients by weight.

Serving size notes the amount per serving, which may be one, or many, tablets.

The % Daily Value is essentially the same as the "U.S. RDA," which used to appear on labels. It tells you the minimum amount of a specific nutrient you need, but not the higher doses often required for therapeutic benefits.

Contact the manufacturer for backup on a product's safety or effectiveness. Buy brands only from a company you trust.

more efficiently utilized by the body than conventional capsules or tablets. In fact, the gel-like substance that acts to delay the release may actually interfere with the absorption of fat-soluble vitamins, such as vitamin A.

And although timed-release versions of niacin (vitamin B_3) may help prevent unpleasant side effects, this formulation is generally not recommended because of the potential risk of liver damage.

Chelated Minerals Chelation is a process in which a mineral is bonded to another substance, or "chelator"—usually an amino acid. This attached substance is supposed to enhance the body's absorption of the mineral. In most cases, there's no proof that chelated minerals are absorbed any better or any quicker than nonchelated minerals. In fact, there is no solid information that any process or added ingredients improve the absorption of vitamins or most minerals.

◆ Standardized Extracts

When herbs are recommended in this book, we often suggest that you look for "standardized extracts." Herbalists and manufacturers use this term to describe the consistency of a product. When creating an herbal supplement, manufacturers can extract the active components from the whole herb. These active ingredients—say, the allicin in garlic or the ginsenosides in ginseng—are then concentrated and made into a supplement (tablets, capsules, tinctures, or liquid extracts). They are standardized in order to supply you with a precise amount of key substances in each dose.

Sometimes, instead of standardized extracts, manufacturers process the whole, or crude, herb. In this case, the whole herb is simply air- or freeze-dried, made into a powder, and then packaged into a supplement—again a capsule, tablet, tincture, liquid extract, or other form.

Whether a standardized extract or the whole herb is better is an ongoing controversy among herbalists. Supporters of whole herb supplements contend that the entire herb may contain still unidentified active ingredients, and that only through ingesting the entire herb can all the benefits be obtained. On the other hand, advocates of standardized extracts argue that the active ingredients in whole herbs can vary greatly depending on where they're grown and how the herbs are harvested and processed. Proponents of standardization say that the only way to be sure you're receiving a consistent amount of active ingredients is by taking only standardized extracts.

Although standardized products are indeed more consistent from batch to batch, this fact doesn't guarantee that they are more effective than whole-herb products. But in many cases, you would have to use a much greater amount of a whole herb to achieve a similar therapeutic effect. More to the point, reliability and consistency can be of great value, particularly when a product proves to be beneficial for a specific disorder.

◆ Multisupplements

Many herbs have traditionally been paired in combination products to enhance their benefits. The most straightforward pairings team herbs with similar effects, such as valerian and chamomile, which both act as sedatives. Other formulas include several herbs that address different symptoms of an ailment, not unlike a combination cold remedy that has one ingredient for congestion, another for sore throat. Still others feature an array of substances touted as antioxidant "cocktails." Supplement manufacturers have also marketed herbs with vitamins and other nutritional supplements such as amino acids.

Some of these combinations can promote health and may also save you money. In addition, you may find that fewer pills are needed. For example, liver detoxifying products called lipotropic combinations often include the nutrients choline, inositol, and

WHEN YOU BUY **STANDARDIZED EXTRACTS**

The amount of an active or main ingredient in a standardized herbal extract is often expressed as a percentage: Milk thistle "standardized to contain 80% silymarin" means that 80% of the extract contains that ingredient. Accordingly, recommendations in this book for most standardized products are given as percentages. For example, a 150 mg dose of milk thistle standardized to contain 80% silymarin contains 120 mg silymarin (150 x .80 = 120).

Sometimes, though, a standardized extract product will simply state the actual amount of active ingredient you're getting (e.g., 120 mg silymarin) rather than listing a percentage. This is fine, too.

methionine, as well as the herb milk thistle—all of which, in a blend, assist liver function. These formulas cost less and are more convenient to take than individual supplements.

In some combination products, however, certain ingredients are present in such small quantities that their therapeutic effect is doubtful. They are there simply to promote the product. So it pays to check the label to determine the amount of each ingredient.

▼ SUPPLEMENT SAFETY

Although supplement manufacturers are prohibited by the Food and Drug Administration (FDA) from making direct claims about curing or treating diseases, the FDA has otherwise given them great leeway, and the safety or effectiveness of a supplement doesn't have to be demonstrated as it does with drugs.

Responsible manufacturers are careful to print instructions about proper use on their labels, but you may encounter many brands that do not supply them. Therefore you need to read the supplement profiles in this book carefully and also keep the following guidelines mind.

◆ *The Proper Amounts*
Dietary supplements are generally safe in the appropriate dosages. But remember that more isn't necessarily better—and sometimes it can be worse. For example, the mineral selenium has many recommended uses, from treating cataracts to preventing cancer. But taking doses even slightly higher than recommended can cause hair loss and other toxic reactions. When using supplements, it's a good idea to avoid high doses, particularly very high ones ("megadoses").

Vitamins and Minerals Most vitamins can be taken in significantly higher doses than their RDAs without producing adverse reactions. However, some fat-soluble vitamins, which are stored in the body rather than excreted, may be toxic at high doses. In particular, overloading on vitamin A or D is dangerous. And although the body naturally excretes extra water-soluable vitamins such as vitamin C, avoid extremely high doses. Toxic reactions can, in fact, occur. Reducing the dosage usually remedies the situation.

Some minerals, taken in large doses or over a long period of time, can block the absorption of other minerals. Zinc, for instance, can hamper the absorption of copper. Also, large amounts of certain minerals have been linked to disease—several studies show that too much iron in men, for example, increases their risk of heart disease. For these reasons, even doctors who believe the RDAs for many vitamins are too low also think that the levels for minerals are generally adequate for optimal health.

Herbs According to reviews by experts in pharmacology and toxicology, serious side effects or toxic reactions associated with herbal medicines are

---

SAFETY GUIDELINES

Because supplements, especially herbs, can have potent primary effects and side effects, keep these points in mind when using them:

• **Shop carefully.** Because there is no independent guarantee of purity or potency, it's your responsibility to select brands with a reputation for quality.

• **Take the recommended dosages.** As with conventional drugs, overdosing with a supplement can have serious consequences. With herbs and nutritional supplements, always start with the lowest dose when a dosage range is given.

• **Monitor your reactions.** At the first sign of an adverse reaction, discontinue using the supplement. Also stop if the herb doesn't seem to be working for you (though give it time—some herbs may take a month or more to have a noticeable effect).

• **Take a break.** Doctors using conventional medications typically recommend "drug holidays" for certain non-life-threatening conditions such as a persistent headache, eczema, or mild depression. The same wisdom applies to supplements: It's best to take them for specified periods, then stop temporarily to see if the condition has improved. If the problem returns, you may need to take the supplement long term as a "maintenance" medication.

• **Avoid risks.** If you have symptoms that indicate a serious problem, don't self-treat it with supplements: See a doctor or other trained health professional. Also ask about interactions with any drugs you are taking.

rare. Still, some once-popular medicinal herbs, such as foxglove and chaparral, are now recognized as toxic. Occasionally, some people exhibit serious allergic reactions to an herb, which may include hives or some other rash, or difficulty breathing.

Furthermore, because no uniform quality control for herbal preparations exists, the chemical composition of an herbal remedy can vary greatly from batch to batch. And it may contain potentially toxic contaminants and other ingredients that can influence side effects or effectiveness. Products that contain standardized extracts may be more reliable than those that don't in terms of getting a proper dose of a particular supplement. But whenever you buy a supplement you still rely on the manufacturer's integrity.

In addition, using some herbs can be risky for people with certain health conditions or for those on particular medications (see pages 182 to 184). Garlic, for example, may intensify the effects of anticoagulant drugs, while licorice—which aids digestive problems and enhances the immune system—can raise blood pressure.

Other herbs may have no immediate adverse effects but may cause side effects or prove harmful when taken over the long term. When using supplements, always follow the dosage recommendations closely. In addition, notify your doctor at once if any serious adverse reactions develop.

▼ QUALITY CONTROL

How do you know what a product actually contains? The best way to find out is to call the manufacturer of a particular supplement and ask how the supplement's potency is assured. You should also check how long the company has been in business. Established supplement manufacturers have a reputation to protect and therefore take measures to ensure that their products contain what is stated on the labels.

You can also ask your doctor or another health professional (such as a dietitian or nutritionist) who uses supplements for recommendations of reliable products.

HOW TO USE THIS BOOK

▼

This book includes profiles of 80 popular supplements, arranged alphabetically from acidophilus to zinc. The preceding pages (6 to 20) provide an overview of the current knowledge about supplements as well as information on the forms they're available in, shopping tips, and safety advice. The appendix features a helpful listing of drug interactions (pages 182 to 184), which you should check if you are taking a conventional prescription or over-the-counter (OTC) medication.

◆ About the Dosages
The dosage suggestions in each profile are the total daily amount that you'll need to treat a disorder. They are based on findings from hundreds of research studies and the clinical experience of the consulting doctors for this book. You may have to adjust these numbers to factor in amounts found in your daily multivitamin or in individual supplements you're already using for other health reasons.

Though we've made every effort to include widely available dosages, the strengths of individual products vary greatly. Many qualified people—health professionals, pharmacists, health-food-store staff—can help you find products with equivalent doses.

◆ Special Exceptions
The recommendations in this book do not apply to pregnant or breast-feeding women, who have specific needs and restrictions, or to children under age 16, whose growth and development vary widely. Individuals in these groups can still benefit from using supplements, but they should always consult a doctor before deciding what supplements to take.

◆ A Final Word
You should talk with your doctor before trying the supplements discussed here, particularly if you have a serious health problem, such as heart disease or diabetes. The book's goal is to inform you about the numerous benefits that can come from taking supplements wisely. This means using them as a complement to—not as a substitute for—responsible medical care.

A to Z
Supplement Profiles

ACIDOPHILUS *(Lactobacillus acidophilus)*

The "friendly" bacteria called acidophilus help create a healthy environment within the gastrointestinal tract. For this reason, taking acidophilus supplements may combat a number of digestive disorders, control recurring vaginal yeast infections, and help the body resist assorted diseases caused by "unfriendly" bacteria.

COMMON USES

■ Treats chronic gastrointestinal tract disorders, such as irritable bowel syndrome, recurrent gas and bloating, and inflammatory bowel disease.

■ Controls vaginal yeast infections.

FORMS

■ Capsule

■ Tablet

■ Liquid

■ Powder

■ Suppository

■ Douche

▼ WHAT IT IS

Some 500 species of bacteria inhabit the digestive tract. Of these, the most beneficial are two strains of *Lactobacilli* bacteria: acidophilus and bifidus. Both are probiotics, meaning they help provide a proper balance of health-promoting bacteria in the intestine. They also manufacture natural antibiotics that are able to kill dangerous microbes.

Yogurt, the traditional source of acidophilus, has been used as an elixir in folk medicine for hundreds, and very possibly thousands, of years. It can be difficult, however, to determine how much acidophilus is really in yogurt.

When using supplements, read labels carefully. A therapeutic form should contain at least 1 billion organisms in each pill; smaller amounts may not be potent enough to have beneficial effects. Acidophilus is sometimes sold in combination with bifidus or with another ingredient that promotes the growth of friendly bacteria called FOS (fructo-oligosaccharides).

▼ WHAT IT DOES

Acidophilus aids in restoring a normal balance of healthy bacteria in the gastrointestinal tract and vagina, thereby helping fight digestive disorders and control vaginal yeast infections. It may contain cancer-fighting agents, and may possibly lower serum cholesterol levels. Acidophilus also supplies certain vitamins, including B_{12}, K, thiamin, and folic acid.

MAJOR BENEFITS

Some studies show that when taken orally or inserted into the vagina as a suppository or douche, acidophilus may prevent or control vaginal yeast infections caused by *Candida albicans*. This property is particularly helpful if you're taking certain types of antibiotics that suppress acidophilus and allow yeast to flourish.

Indeed, acidophilus may be especially useful for anyone taking antibiotics to treat an infection. A healthy colon should contain about 85% *Lactobacilli* (including acidophilus and bifidus) and 14% coliform bacteria

⧯ ALERT ⧯

SIDE EFFECTS
• Ingested in large quantities, acidophilus may cause diarrhea or other gastrointestinal complaints.

• Prolonged douching with acidophilus can irritate the vagina.

CAUTION
• If you have a vaginal infection for the first time, see your doctor before treating it yourself. Acidophilus is useful against the yeast *Candida albicans*, but has little effect on other types of vaginal problems and may worsen their symptoms.

• **Reminder:** If you have a medical condition, talk to your doctor before taking supplements.

(including healthy types of E. coli and other bacterial strains). In many people (and particularly those on antibiotics) these counts can be upset, causing flatulence, diarrhea, constipation, and poor absorption of nutrients. Acidophilus creates an inhospitable environment for harmful types of E. coli bacteria, as well as for salmonella, streptococcus, and many other strains of bacteria that can be dangerous or even life-threatening.

ADDITIONAL BENEFITS

Acidophilus can reduce the symptoms of inflammatory bowel disease, a chronic inflammation of the intestines. Along with a high-fiber diet, acidophilus contributes to overall colon health, which is necessary to help avert diverticulosis, a disorder in which the mucous lining of the colon bulges into the colon wall and creates small sacs (diverticula). Acidophilus may also relieve diarrhea triggered by irritable bowel syndrome and replenish beneficial intestinal microorganisms that diarrhea flushes out of the body.

Moreover, studies in animals suggest that acidophilus may be valuable in combating some cancers. When given to patients surgically treated for bladder cancer, acidophilus helped prevent the recurrence of single tumors. This result may have occurred because acidophilus prevents harmful bacteria from creating cancer-causing substances

when the bacteria react with foods. Acidophilus may also lower blood cholesterol levels. Certain strains of these bacteria absorb cholesterol in the intestine before it reaches the arteries and does damage.

▼ HOW TO TAKE IT

DOSAGE

To make a vaginal douche: Mix 2 teaspoons of acidophilus/bifidus powder in a quart of warm water; use twice a day for up to 10 days to restore normal bacterial growth.
To promote intestinal health: Mix acidophilus/bifidus powder in water and drink; see label for exact dose. In capsule form, take one or two, each containing at least 1 billion live organisms, one to three times daily. For other forms, follow the directions on the label.

GUIDELINES FOR USE

• Douching is best reserved for treating vaginal yeast infections, or for those times you are taking antibiotics.

• When using acidophilus orally, take it half an hour to an hour before eating.

• If you are on antibiotics, do not take your prescription medication at the same time of day as the acidophilus. And continue the acidophilus even after you finish the antibiotics.

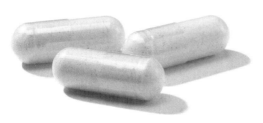

SHOPPING HINTS

■ Acidophilus products should say they contain "live cultures" or "active cultures." Be sure to check for an expiration date.

■ Whatever form you purchase, store it in a cool, dry place, such as the refrigerator. Heat can easily kill live acidophilus; freezing temperatures can as well.

LATEST FINDINGS

■ A recent study showed that eating yogurt containing live acidophilus greatly reduced the recurrence of vaginal yeast infections. The women in the study ate 8 ounces of yogurt every day for six months. Researchers theorize that additional acidophilus bacteria grow in the vaginal canal, which bolsters the normal *Lactobacilli* flora but leaves no room for the growth of yeast.

■ When used in a recent study of patients undergoing cancer radiation treatments, acidophilus prevented the diarrhea that is a typical side effect of this therapy. Patients drank a fermented milk product containing live acidophilus bacteria daily.

DID YOU KNOW?

Because high heat will kill acidophilus cultures, some commercial yogurt manufacturers add the active cultures after the pasteurization process is completed.

ALOE VERA *(Aloe vera, A. barbadensis, A. vulgaris)*

Since the reign of Cleopatra in ancient Egypt, the cool, soothing gel from inside the fleshy leaf of the aloe vera plant has been gently applied to treat skin problems, ranging from burns and minor wounds to itchy insect bites. This clear gel is also the basis of aloe vera juice, which can calm digestive complaints.

COMMON USES

Applied topically

■ Heals minor burns, cuts and abrasions, insect bites and stings, welts, small skin ulcers, and frostbite.

■ Relieves the itch of shingles (herpes zoster).

■ May help clear up warts.

Taken internally

■ Soothes ulcers, heartburn, and other digestive complaints.

FORMS

■ Cream/Ointment
■ Fresh herb/Gel
■ Liquid/Juice
■ Capsule
■ Softgel

▼ WHAT IT IS

A succulent in the Lily family, aloe vera has fleshy leaves that provide a gel widely used as a topical treatment for skin problems—a practice dating back to at least 1500 B.C., when Egyptian healers described it in their treatises.

The plant is native to the Cape of Good Hope and grows wild in much of Africa and Madagascar; commercial growers cultivate it in the Caribbean, the Mediterranean, Japan, and the United States.

▼ WHAT IT DOES

Scientists aren't exactly sure how aloe vera works, but they have identified many of its active ingredients. Rich in anti-inflammatory substances, the gel contains a gummy material that acts as a soothing emollient, as well as brady-kininase, a compound that helps treat pain and reduce swelling, and magnesium lactate, which quells itching.

Aloe vera also dilates the tiny blood vessels known as capillaries, allowing more blood to get to an injury and thus speeding up the healing process. In addition, some studies show that it destroys, or at least inhibits, a number of bacteria, viruses, and fungi.

MAJOR BENEFITS

Aloe vera gel is particularly helpful when applied to damaged skin. It aids in the healing of first-degree burns, sunburn, minor skin wounds, and even painful shingles by relieving pain and reducing itching. The gel also provides an airproof moisturizing barrier, so that wounds do not dry out. Furthermore, aloe vera's capillary-dilating properties increase blood circulation, speeding the regeneration of skin and relieving mild cases of frostbite. The gel's anti-viral effects may promote the healing of warts as well.

Though effective against minor cuts and abrasions, aloe vera may not be a good choice for more serious, infected wounds. In a study of 21 new mothers who were hospitalized in Los Angeles with infected cesarean-section wounds, applying the herbal aloe vera gel actually increased the length of time—from

  ALERT

SIDE EFFECTS

• Topical aloe vera is very safe. In rare cases, some people get a mild, allergic skin reaction with itching or rash; simply discontinue use.

• Aloe vera juice, however, may contain small amounts of the laxative ingredient in aloe latex because of poor processing. If you experience cramping, diarrhea, or loose stools, stop taking the juice immediately. Never take aloe vera juice if you are pregnant or breast-feeding.

CAUTION

• Don't confuse aloe vera with the bitter yellow aloe latex, which is sold as a laxative and can cause severe cramping and diarrhea. Pregnant or breast-feeding women in particular should avoid aloe latex.

• **Reminder:** If you have a medical condition, talk to your doctor before taking supplements.

53 to 83 days–that it took for the abdominal wounds to heal.

ADDITIONAL BENEFITS

Aloe vera gel is also used to make a juice that may be taken internally for inflammatory digestive disorders, including ulcers and heartburn. However, there's very little research on its internal use.

In Japan, purified aloe vera compounds have been found to inhibit stomach secretions and lesions. In one study, aloe vera juice cured 17 of 18 patients with peptic ulcers, but, unfortunately, there was no comparison group taking a placebo. A U.S. commercial lab is currently conducting trials with an aloe-derived compound as a treatment for people with ulcerative colitis–a type of inflammatory bowel disease.

Other studies are exploring aloe vera's effectiveness as a possible antiviral and immune-boosting agent for people with AIDS; as a treatment for leukemia and other types of cancer; and as a therapy to help those with diabetes manage the demands of their disease.

▼ HOW TO TAKE IT

DOSAGE

For external use: Liberally apply aloe vera gel or cream to injured skin as needed or desired.

For internal use: Take one-half to three-quarters of a cup of aloe vera juice three times a day; or take one or two capsules as directed on the label.

GUIDELINES FOR USE

• Topically, aloe vera gel can be applied repeatedly, especially in the case of burns. Just rub it on the affected area, let it dry, and reapply when needed. Fresh gel from a live leaf is the most potent (and economical) form of the herb. If you have an aloe vera plant, cut off several inches from a leaf, then slice the cutting lengthwise. Spread the gel from the center of the leaf onto the affected area.

• For internal use, take aloe vera juice between meals. Another form of aloe called aloe latex, a yellow extract from the inner leaf, is a powerful laxative and should be used only sparingly under a doctor's care.

The gel-filled leaf of the aloe vera plant is the source of healing pills and juice.

SHOPPING HINTS

■ When buying aloe products, be sure aloe vera is near the top of the ingredients list. Creams and ointments should contain at least 20% aloe vera. For internal use, look for juice that contains at least 98% aloe vera and no aloin or aloe-emodin.

■ The International Aloe Science Council, a voluntary certification program, provides the "IASC-certified" seal to products that use certified raw ingredients and process them according to standard guidelines. Look for this seal, especially when you are purchasing aloe vera juice.

LATEST FINDINGS

■ Add another potential use for aloe vera gel: treating the inflammatory skin condition psoriasis. A study of 60 people with long-standing psoriasis found that applying aloe to skin lesions three times a day for eight months led to significant improvement in 83% of the patients, versus only 6% in those who used a placebo.

DID YOU KNOW?

Aloe vera makes a soothing bath, which is especially helpful for sunburn. Just add a cup or two of the juice to a tub of lukewarm water.

ALPHA-LIPOIC ACID

This relatively recent addition to the supplement scene has shown great promise in treating nerve damage in people with diabetes. Alpha-lipoic acid also appears to protect the liver and brain cells, prevent cataracts, and serve as a powerful general antioxidant because it's easily absorbed by most tissues in the body.

COMMON USES

■ Helps treat numbness, tingling, and other symptoms of nerve damage in people with diabetes or other nerve-related conditions.

■ Protects the liver from damage due to hepatitis, alcohol abuse, or exposure to toxic chemicals.

■ Aids in preventing cataracts.

■ May help preserve memory in Alzheimer's disease.

■ Serves as a high-potency antioxidant and possible immune booster, combating a wide range of disorders, including psoriasis, fibromyalgia, and AIDS.

FORMS

■ Tablet
■ Capsule

▼ WHAT IT IS

In the 1950s scientists discovered that versatile alpha-lipoic acid (also known as thioctic acid or simply lipoic acid) worked with enzymes throughout the body to speed the processes involved in energy production. More recently, in the late 1980s, researchers found that alpha-lipoic acid can be a powerful antioxidant as well, neutralizing naturally occurring, highly reactive molecules called free radicals that can damage cells.

Although the body manufactures it in minute amounts, alpha-lipoic acid is mainly present in foods such as spinach, meats (especially liver), and brewer's yeast. It's difficult, however, to obtain therapeutic amounts of this vitaminlike substance through diet alone. Instead, many nutritional experts recommend using supplements to get the full benefits of alpha-lipoic acid.

▼ WHAT IT DOES

Alpha-lipoic acid affects nearly every cell in the body. It assists all of the B vitamins (including thiamin, riboflavin, pantothenic acid, and niacin) in converting carbohydrates, protein, and fats found in foods into energy that the body can store and later use.

Alpha-lipoic acid is a cell-protecting antioxidant that may help the body recycle other antioxidants, such as vitamins C and E, boosting their potency. Thanks to its unique chemical properties, alpha-lipoic acid is easily absorbed by most tissues in the body, including the brain, nerves, and liver, making it valuable for treating a wide range of different ailments.

MAJOR BENEFITS
One of alpha-lipoic acid's primary uses is to treat nerve damage, including diabetic neuropathy, a dangerous long-term complication of diabetes that causes pain and loss of feeling in the limbs. The nerve condition may be partly due to free-radical damage to nerve cells caused by runaway levels of sugar (glucose) in the blood. Alpha-lipoic acid may play a role in countering such nerve damage because of its antioxidant effects.

ALERT

SIDE EFFECTS
• Alpha-lipoic acid appears to be very safe, and there have been no reports of serious side effects in people taking it.

• Occasionally, the supplement may produce mild gastrointestinal upset, and in rare cases, allergic skin rashes have occurred. If side effects appear, lower the dose or discontinue using the supplement.

CAUTION
• For people with diabetes, the use of alpha-lipoic acid may require a change in insulin or other medications.

• **Reminder:** If you have a medical condition, talk to your doctor before taking supplements.

In addition, alpha-lipoic acid can help people with diabetes respond to insulin, the hormone that regulates glucose. In a study of 74 people with type 2 diabetes who were given 600 mg or more of alpha-lipoic acid daily, all benefited from lowered glucose levels.

Studies in animals also show that alpha-lipoic acid increases blood flow to the nerves and enhances the conduction of nerve impulses. These effects may make alpha-lipoic acid suitable for the treatment of numbness, tingling, and other symptoms of nerve damage from any cause, not just diabetes.

Alpha-lipoic acid also assists the liver, protecting it against damage from free radicals and helping it clear toxins from the body. It is therefore sometimes used to treat hepatitis, cirrhosis, and other liver ailments, as well as in cases of poisoning—by lead or other heavy metals, or by hazardous industrial chemicals such as carbon tetrachloride.

ADDITIONAL BENEFITS
Alpha-lipoic acid may have other potential uses, although more research is needed. Some compelling studies in animals show that it can prevent cataracts from forming. Additional animal experiments suggest that it may improve memory (making it potentially beneficial against Alzheimer's disease, for example) and protect brain cells against damage caused by an insufficient blood supply to the brain (the result of surgery or stroke, for example).

Some evidence indicates alpha-lipoic acid, through its antioxidant capacities, can suppress viral reproduction. In one study, alpha-lipoic acid supplements were shown to boost immune and liver function in a majority of patients infected with AIDS. It may also help in the fight against cancer, especially the forms of the disease thought to be related to free-radical damage.

Finally, as part of a general high-potency antioxidant formula, alpha-lipoic acid may prove effective against disorders ranging from fibromyalgia to psoriasis, which may be aggravated, in part, by free-radical damage.

▼ HOW TO TAKE IT

DOSAGE
To treat specific disorders:
Alpha-lipoic acid is usually taken in doses of 100 to 200 mg three times a day.
For general antioxidant support: Lower doses of 50 to 150 mg a day may be used.

GUIDELINES FOR USE
• Alpha-lipoic acid can be taken with or without food. No major adverse effects have been reported.

• Single antioxidants such as alpha-lipoic acid are no longer recommended for use at high doses. Combination products are safer, more convenient, and less costly.

SHOPPING HINTS
■ Alpha-lipoic acid can be purchased as an individual supplement or part of a general antioxidant booster (with vitamins C, E, and others). Look for it on the ingredients list; it may also be called thioctic acid. Blends are probably the most effective way to take any antioxidant.

LATEST FINDINGS
■ In a trial at multiple medical centers, 328 people with diabetic nerve damage were given 100 mg, 600 mg, or 1,200 mg of alpha-lipoic acid a day over a three-week period. Compared with other groups, patients receiving 600 mg reported the most significant reduction in pain and numbness.

■ Alpha-lipoic acid may also benefit the 25% of diabetes sufferers who are at risk of sudden death from nerve-related heart damage. After four months of taking 800 mg of alpha-lipoic acid a day, these patients showed a notable improvement in their heart function tests.

■ A study of aged mice indicated that alpha-lipoic acid improved long-term memory, possibly by preventing free-radical damage to brain cells.

DID YOU KNOW?
Doctors have used an injectable form of alpha-lipoic acid to save the lives of people who mistakenly ate poisonous amanita mushrooms picked in the wild.

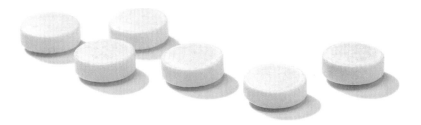

AMINO ACIDS

The protein in food and in your body is a combination of chemical units called amino acids. A diet lacking even one amino acid can have a negative effect on your health. Supplements may be needed to help your body work more efficiently and to treat medical conditions ranging from heart disease to cold sores.

COMMON USES

- Treat heart disease.
- Lower blood pressure.
- Boost immune function.
- Improve some nerve disorders.

FORMS

- Capsule
- Tablet
- Liquid
- Powder

▼ WHAT IT IS

Every cell in the body needs and uses amino acids. Your body breaks down the protein from foods into its individual amino acids, which are then recombined to create the specific types of proteins the body requires. (Each cell, in fact, is programmed to produce exactly the right combination for its particular needs.)

There are two types of amino acids: nonessential and essential. The body can manufacture nonessential amino acids, but must obtain essential amino acids from the foods you eat.

Nonessential amino acids include alanine, arginine, asparagine, aspartic acid, cysteine, glutamic acid, glutamine, glycine, proline, serine, taurine, and tyrosine. Essential amino acids include histidine, isoleucine, leucine, lysine, methionine, phenylalanine, threonine, tryptophan, and valine.

▼ WHAT IT DOES

Amino acids are needed to maintain and repair muscles, tendons, skin, ligaments, organs, glands, nails, and hair. They also aid in the production of hormones (such as insulin), neurotransmitters (message-carrying chemicals within the brain), various body fluids, and enzymes that trigger bodily functions. When even one amino acid is lacking, serious health problems will eventually occur.

Though the major cause of an amino acid deficiency is a poor diet (particularly one low in protein), amino acids may also be affected by infection, trauma, stress, medications, age, and chemical imbalances within the body.

Nutritionally oriented doctors often give blood tests to determine whether a patient has a deficiency. Amino acid supplements can compensate for such deficiencies and can also be taken therapeutically (even when patients aren't deficient) for a wide variety of health problems.

MAJOR BENEFITS

Different amino acids (and their byproducts) are very effective in the treatment of heart disease. Highly concentrated in the cells of the heart

ALERT

SIDE EFFECTS
- Amino acid supplements have no side effects as long as they are taken in the recommended amounts. High doses of certain amino acids, however, may be toxic and produce nausea, vomiting, or diarrhea.

CAUTION
- Pregnant women or anyone with liver or kidney disease should consult a doctor about using amino acid supplements.

- **Reminder:** If you have a medical condition, talk to your doctor before taking supplements.

muscle, carnitine—a substance similar to an amino acid that the body produces from lysine—strengthens the heart, helps those with congestive heart failure, and can improve the chances of surviving a heart attack. Because it is also involved in fat metabolism, carnitine may help lower high levels of trigylcerides (blood fats related to cholesterol).

The nonessential amino acid arginine reduces the risk of heart attack and stroke by widening blood vessels and lowering blood pressure; it eases the symptoms and pains of angina as well. Taurine treats congestive heart failure and lowers high blood pressure by balancing the blood's ratio of sodium to potassium and by regulating excessive activity of the central nervous system.

N-acetylcysteine (NAC), a by-product of the amino acid cysteine that's better absorbed than cysteine, stimulates the body's production of antioxidants and may be an antioxidant itself. As such, it aids in repairing cell damage and boosting the immune system. NAC also thins the mucus of chronic bronchitis and has been used to protect the liver in overdoses of acetaminophen (Tylenol). It may also be of value for disorders involving damage to brain or nerve cells, such as multiple sclerosis.

ADDITIONAL BENEFITS
Concentrated in the cells of the digestive tract, glutamine can help heal ulcers and soothe irritable bowel syndrome and diverticulosis. By enhancing the production of certain brain chemicals, taurine may be a boon to people with epilepsy. It's also a key element in bile and may prevent gallstones. People with diabetes can also benefit from taurine because it facilitates the body's use of insulin.

Carnitine feeds the muscles by making it possible for them to burn fat for energy. Lysine is one of the most effective treatments for cold sores and is also useful for shingles and canker sores. (Arginine, on the other hand, can trigger cold sore or genital herpes outbreaks.)

▼ HOW TO TAKE IT

DOSAGE
For the recommended dosage of individual amino acids, follow label directions on the package.

When using any individual amino acid for longer than one month, take it with a mixed amino acid complex—a supplement that contains a variety of amino acids—to be sure you are receiving adequate, balanced amounts of all the amino acids.

GUIDELINES FOR USE
• Amino acid supplements are more effective when they don't have to compete with the amino acids in high-protein foods. Take the supplements at least an hour and a half before or after meals (first thing in the morning or at bedtime may be best).

• Individual amino acid supplements should not be used for longer than three months, unless you are under the supervision of a doctor familiar with their use.

• Take mixed amino acid supplements on an empty stomach and not at the same time of day that you take the individual supplement.

SHOPPING HINTS
■ On supplement labels, amino acids are often prefaced by an L (L-carnitine, for example) or by a D. Buy the L forms: They most closely resemble the amino acids in the body. (One exception: D-L phenylalanine may be useful for chronic pain.)

LATEST FINDINGS
■ Carnitine improved the symptoms of intermittent claudication (leg pain caused by the blockage of large arteries in legs) in 73% of people taking a specialized form of this amino acid, according to a study from Italy. Often people with this condition can't walk very far. L-carnitine in doses up to 2,000 mg a day increased the distance the participants could walk without pain.

■ Researchers at Stanford University found that arginine supplements may reduce the tendency for blood platelets to stick to each other and to artery walls, thereby preventing clots that cause heart attacks and strokes. Arginine particularly benefits people with high cholesterol because they tend to have stickier platelets than those with normal cholesterol.

ASTRAGALUS *(Astragalus membranaceous)*

For more than 2,000 years, astragalus has been an integral part of traditional medicine in China, where it is used to balance the life force, or *qi*. Because of its powerful effect on the immune system, this herb is particularly valuable for fighting disease and for dealing with the aftereffects of cancer treatments.

COMMON USES

- Enhances immunity.
- Helps fight respiratory infections.
- Bolsters the immune system in people undergoing cancer treatment.

FORMS

- Tablet
- Capsule
- Liquid extract
- Dried herb/Tea

▼ WHAT IT IS

Astragalus contains a variety of compounds that stimulate the body's immune system, and in China this native plant has long been used both to treat disease and to prevent it.

Botanically, astragalus is related to licorice and the pea. And although its sweet-smelling pale yellow blossoms and delicate structure give the plant a frail appearance, it is actually a very hardy species.

Medicinally, the herb's most important part is its root. The plant is harvested when it is four to seven years old; its flat, yellowish roots resemble wide popsicle sticks or tongue depressors. (The Chinese name for astragalus, *huang qi*, means "yellow leader," a testament both to its color and to its importance as a therapeutic herb.) Astragalus root is loaded with health-promoting substances, including polysaccharides, a class of carbohydrates that appear to be responsible for the herb's immune-boosting effects.

▼ WHAT IT DOES

A tonic in the truest sense of the word, astragalus seems to enhance overall health by improving a person's resistance to disease, increasing stamina and vitality, and promoting general well-being. It also acts as an antioxidant, helping the body correct or prevent cell damage caused by free radicals. It may have antiviral and antibiotic properties as well.

A distinct benefit of astragalus is that it can be safely used with conventional medicine and does not interfere with any standard treatment.

PREVENTION

This herb is particularly effective in fighting off colds, the flu, bronchitis, and sinus infections because it keeps viruses from gaining a foothold in the respiratory system. Like echinacea, astragalus can squash germs at the first sign of symptoms.

And if an illness does develop, astragalus can shorten its duration and often reduce its severity. People who frequently suffer from respiratory problems should consider using astragalus on a regular basis to prevent

 ALERT

SIDE EFFECTS
- Remarkably, even after thousands of years of use in China, there are few (if any) negative reports about taking astragalus. The herb appears to have no side effects of any kind.

CAUTION
- Pregnant women should consult with their doctor before using this herb.

- **Reminder:** If you have a medical condition, talk to your doctor before taking supplements.

recurrences. It also appears to help minimize the health-damaging effects of excessive stress.

ADDITIONAL BENEFITS

Astragalus is widely used in China to rebuild the immune system of people undergoing radiation or chemotherapy for cancer; in fact, this practice is gaining popularity in the West as well. The herb is especially valuable because it increases the body's production of T cells, macrophages, natural killer cells, interferon, and other immune cells.

Astragalus may also protect bone marrow from the immune-suppressing effects of chemotherapy, radiation, toxins, and viruses. The herb, with its immune-stimulating action, might be a treatment possibility for people infected with HIV, the virus that causes AIDS.

In addition, astragalus widens blood vessels and increases blood flow, which makes it useful in controlling excessive perspiration (such as night sweats) and lowering blood pressure. Research has also shown that astragalus can have beneficial effects on the heart.

▼ HOW TO TAKE IT

DOSAGE

For strengthening the immune system: Take 200 mg of astragalus once or twice a day for three weeks; then alternate, in three-week stints, with the herbs echinacea, cat's claw, and pau d'arco.
For acute bronchitis: Take 200 mg four times a day until the symptoms ease. Always try to choose a product that contains a standardized extract of astragalus with 0.5% glucosides and 70% polysaccharides.

GUIDELINES FOR USE

• The herb astragalus can be taken at any time during the day, with or without food.

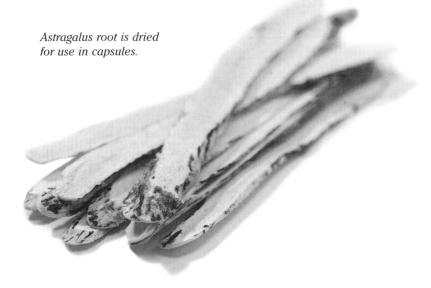

Astragalus root is dried for use in capsules.

FACTS & TIPS

■ In China, dried astragalus root is often sliced and added to soup to sweeten the flavor. Before the soup is eaten, the slices are removed because they're tough and hard to chew.

■ To help enhance its healing properties, astragalus is often combined with herbs such as ginseng, licorice, and echinacea.

LATEST FINDINGS

Two separate studies conducted in China showed that astragalus can benefit people with heart disease.

■ The first study revealed that if astragalus was taken within 36 hours of a heart attack, it could bolster the functioning of the heart's left ventricle, the chamber that pumps oxygen-rich blood throughout the body.

■ The second study examined whether astragalus could lessen chest pain (angina). The herb was compared to nifedipine, a prescription medication commonly used to treat this condition. The study found that astragalus produced better results than the drug.

DID YOU KNOW?

Several North American species of astragalus are highly poisonous to livestock; they're commonly called "locoweed." These New World varieties, however, are very different from the ancient Chinese form of astragalus used medicinally.

BEE PRODUCTS

Although over the years many intriguing claims have been made for the natural healing powers of bee products, there is little scientific evidence to support most of them. Yet bee pollen, royal jelly, and propolis remain popular nutritional supplements, and they continue to be the subject of ongoing research studies.

COMMON USES
- May help hay fever symptoms.
- Aids in healing skin abrasions.

FORMS
- Tablet
- Capsule
- Softgel
- Liquid
- Powder/Granules
- Cream
- Lozenge
- Dried and fresh pollen

▼ WHAT IT IS

There are three types of bee products available in health-food stores: bee pollen, propolis, and royal jelly. The most familiar of these is bee pollen. After the bees gather pollen from plants, they compress it into pellets, which beekeepers then collect from the hives. (A second type of pollen, also sold as bee pollen, is collected directly from plants, not from bees at all.) Bee pollen contains protein, B vitamins, carbohydrates, and various enzymes.

Propolis (also called bee glue) is a sticky resin that bees collect from the buds of pine trees and use to repair cracks in their hives. Then there's royal jelly, a milky-white substance produced by the salivary glands of worker bees as a food source for the queen bee.

The specialized nutritional content of royal jelly may account for the fertility, large size, and increased longevity of the queen.

▼ WHAT IT DOES

Bee products, especially bee pollen, have been touted as virtual cure-alls. Proponents assert that, among other things, these products slow aging, improve athletic performance, boost immunity, contribute to weight loss, fight bacteria, and alleviate the symptoms of allergies and hay fever.

Although bee pollen shows some promise in treating allergies, and propolis may be an effective salve for cuts and bruises, the scant research that has been conducted does not support the extravagant claims generally made for bee products.

MAJOR BENEFITS
Bee pollen seems to help prevent the sneezing, runny nose, watery eyes, and other symptoms of seasonal pollen allergies. Some scientists believe that ingesting small amounts of pollen can desensitize an individual to its allergenic compounds, much as allergy shots do. Because your body produces antibodies when exposed to even a tiny amount of pollen, your immune system then "remembers" it, preventing an extreme reaction that causes classic allergy symptoms.

 ALERT

SIDE EFFECTS
- Because some individuals will have an allergic reaction to bee pollen, begin with a small amount so you can determine if it will have an adverse effect on you. Watch for hives, itchy throat, skin flushing, wheezing, or headache. Discontinue use immediately if any of these reactions occur.

CAUTION
- People with asthma or allergies to bee stings should be very careful when using bee products; they should avoid royal jelly entirely.

- **Reminder:** If you have a medical condition, talk to your doctor before taking supplements.

Testing of this theory is under way and until results are available, there appears to be no harm for most people in trying bee pollen. Various advocates maintain that to get the full anti-allergy benefit, you need to use bee pollen that comes from a local source, which will desensitize you to the specific pollens in your own environment.

ADDITIONAL BENEFITS
Bee propolis may play some role as a skin softener or wound healer. Research has shown that though propolis contains antibacterial compounds, these are not as effective as standard antibiotics or over-the-counter antibiotic ointments in fighting infection.

Because royal jelly enhances the growth, fertility, and longevity of queen bees, many people think that it will do the same thing for humans. However, there's no evidence to support this view, so there appears to be little reason to use royal jelly.

▼ HOW TO TAKE IT

DOSAGE
The amount of bee pollen needed to relieve allergy symptoms varies from person to person. In general, start with a few granules a day and increase the dose gradually until you're up to 1 to 3 rounded teaspoons a day.

GUIDELINES FOR USE
• Prior to hay fever season, start taking very small amounts of bee pollen each day—a few granules or a portion of a tablet. If you don't suffer any adverse reaction (see Alert box opposite), slowly increase your dosage every few days until you experience relief from your allergy symptoms.

• Have bee pollen supplements with plenty of water; you can also mix dried or fresh pollen with juice or sprinkle it over food.

CASE HISTORY

A Killer Drink
From childhood, Jerry H., a bond trader, knew he was deathly allergic to bee stings and avoided the buzzing, venom-carrying insects like the plague. But, surprisingly, it was a health-food drink that almost killed him.

As was his habit, Jerry often skipped lunch while he worked and then stopped at his favorite health-food store on the way home for a quick pick-me-up.

On the fateful day, he took the advice of an enthusiastic clerk and ordered "The Kitchen Sink Smoothie," a special new yogurt drink. Little did he realize it contained a generous scoop of some "energizing" bee product in addition to the touted ginseng, spirulina, and wheatgrass.

The last thing Jerry remembers about his close brush with oblivion was "putting the glass to my lips." When he awoke, he found himself in an intensive care unit recovering from anaphylactic shock. His advice to others with a bee allergy: "Watch those healthy drinks. They can be lethal."

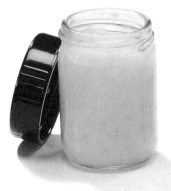
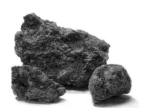
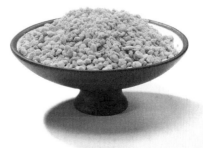

The three types of bee products on the market are royal jelly (left), propolis (center), and bee pollen (right).

BETA-CAROTENE

Once considered just a potent source of vitamin A, beta-carotene has recently gained prominence as a disease-fighting substance. Today, experts think that beta-carotene—along with a number of related nutrients called carotenoids—may protect against such serious illnesses as heart disease and cancer.

COMMON USES

■ Acts as a preventive for cancer and heart disease.

■ May reverse some precancerous conditions.

■ Has cell-protecting properties that may aid in the treatment of a wide variety of ailments from Alzheimer's disease to male infertility.

FORMS

■ Capsule
■ Tablet
■ Softgel
■ Liquid

▼ WHAT IT IS

Beta-carotene is part of a larger team of nutrients known as carotenoids, which are the yellow-orange pigments found in fruits and vegetables (see page 44). Because the body converts it to vitamin A, beta-carotene is sometimes called provitamin A. However, beta-carotene provides many additional benefits besides supplying the body with that vitamin.

▼ WHAT IT DOES

An immune system booster and powerful antioxidant, beta-carotene helps neutralizes the free radicals that can damage cells and promote disease. By acting directly on cells, it combats—and may even reverse—some disorders. It appears to be most effective when combined with other carotenoids.

PREVENTION

Beta-carotene is a celebrated soldier in the war on heart disease. Results from a survey of more than 300 doctors enrolled in the Harvard University Physicians' Health Study revealed that taking 50 mg (85,000 IU) of beta-carotene a day cut the risk of heart attack, stroke, and all cardiovascular deaths in half. Other studies have shown that it can prevent LDL ("bad") cholesterol from damaging the heart and coronary vessels. High levels of beta-carotene may also offer protection against cancers of the lung, digestive tract, bladder, breast, and prostate.

MAJOR BENEFITS

Acting as an antioxidant, beta-carotene has reversed some precancerous conditions, particularly those affecting the skin, mucous membranes, lungs, mouth, throat, stomach, colon, prostate, cervix, and uterus. Further, it has been shown to inhibit the growth of abnormal cells, strengthen the immune system, fortify cell membranes, and increase communication among cells.

One hint of concern did arise, however, about beta-carotene's cancer-fighting benefits. In the early 1990s, landmark studies in Finland and the United States found that male smokers taking beta-carotene supplements had an increased risk of lung cancer. Though some found the studies flawed, many experts caution smokers to maintain adequate beta-carotene levels through

 ALERT

CAUTION

• Consult your physician before using beta-carotene if you have a sluggish thyroid (hypothyroidism), kidney or liver disease, or an eating disorder.

• Many experts recommend that smokers, particularly those who consume large amounts of alcohol, avoid beta-carotene supplements.

• Don't take more than 50,000 IU of beta-carotene daily.

• **Reminder:** If you have a medical condition, talk to your doctor before taking supplements.

natural food sources, not through dietary supplements.

ADDITIONAL BENEFITS

As an antioxidant, beta-carotene may be helpful for a wide range of additional ailments, including Alzheimer's disease, chronic fatigue syndrome, male infertility, fibromyalgia, psoriasis, and a number of vision disorders.

▼ HOW MUCH YOU NEED

There is no RDA for beta-carotene, although about 10,000 IU meets the RDA for vitamin A. Higher doses are needed, however, to provide the full antioxidant and immune-boosting effects. Recent findings (including the Finnish smokers study), however, showed that megadoses may do more harm than good. For this reason, it's advisable to limit your upper daily intake to no more than 50,000 IU daily.

IF YOU GET TOO LITTLE

Signs of a beta-carotene deficiency are similar to those of inadequate vitamin A: poor night vision, dry skin, increased risk of infection, and the formation of precancerous cells. A deficiency may also increase your risk of cancer and heart disease. However, vitamin A deficiencies are rare: Even if you don't eat fruits and vegetables or take supplements, you can still meet your vitamin A needs with eggs, fortified milk, or other foods that supply it.

IF YOU GET TOO MUCH

For the most part, the body discards what beta-carotene it doesn't process. If you ingest high levels in foods or supplements (more than 100,000 IU a day), your palms and soles may turn a harmless orange tone, which will disappear when you lower the dose.

▼ HOW TO TAKE IT

DOSAGE

Beta-carotene is probably most effective when combined with other carotenoids in a mixed-carotenoid formula. Most people benefit from one dose daily of a mixed-carotenoid supplement that provides 25,000 IU vitamin A activity. If you are at particularly high risk for cancer or heart disease, consider increasing your dose to two mixed-carotenoid pills daily.

GUIDELINES FOR USE

• Take supplements with meals.

• No adverse effects have been noted in pregnant or nursing women taking up to 50,000 IU a day.

▼ OTHER SOURCES

Carrots are a rich source of beta-carotene, as are other yellow, orange, and red fruits and vegetables, from sweet potatoes to cantaloupe. Green vegetables, such as broccoli, spinach, or lettuce, are also beneficial—the darker the green, the more beta-carotene they contain.

SHOPPING HINTS

■ Purchase beta-carotene in combination with other carotenoids, such as lycopene, alpha-carotene, cryptoxanthin, zeaxanthin, and lutein. These combination formulas are a safe, effective, and thrifty way to boost your body's antioxidant levels.

LATEST FINDINGS

■ Beta-carotene may help protect against many types of cancer—but in smokers, it may actually increase the risk of lung cancer. Recent studies show that this surprising effect seems strongest in men who smoke at least 20 cigarettes daily and increases further when alcohol intake is "above average." (Interestingly, former smokers do not appear to be at heightened risk.) One theory is that smokers generally have low vitamin C levels, and this imbalance causes beta-carotene to heighten, rather than decrease, free-radical formation.

DID YOU KNOW?

You'd have to eat more than a pound of fresh cantaloupe to get the beta-carotene in one 25,000 IU capsule.

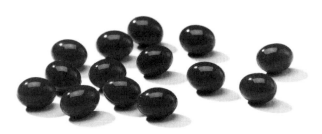

BILBERRY *(Vaccinium myrtillus)*

During World War II, British RAF pilots noted the curious fact that their night vision improved after they had eaten bilberry preserves. Their anecdotal reports sparked scientific research on this herb, which today is used to treat a wide range of visual disorders—from night blindness to cataracts—as well as other complaints.

COMMON USES

- Maintains healthy vision and improves night vision and poor visual adaptation to bright light.
- Treats a wide array of eye disorders, including diabetic retinopathy, cataracts, and macular degeneration.
- Relieves varicose veins and hemorrhoids.

FORMS

- Tablet
- Capsule
- Softgel
- Liquid extract
- Dried herb/Tea

▼ WHAT IT IS

Although the fruit of the bilberry bush has been enjoyed since prehistoric times, its first recorded medicinal use was in the sixteenth century. Historically, dried berry or leaf preparations were recommended for a variety of conditions, including scurvy (a disease caused by a severe vitamin C deficiency), urinary tract infections, and kidney stones.

A relative of the American blueberry, bilberry is a short, shrubby perennial that grows in the forests and wooded meadows of northern Europe. Bushes of these sweet blue-black berries are also found in western Asia and the Rocky Mountains of North America.

The medically active components in the ripe fruit consist primarily of flavonoid compounds known as anthocyanosides. Accordingly, the modern medicinal form of bilberry is an extract containing a highly concentrated amount of these compounds.

▼ WHAT IT DOES

Many of the medicinal qualities of bilberry derive from its major constituents, anthocyanosides, which are potent antioxidants. These compounds help counteract cell damage caused by unstable oxygen molecules called free radicals.

MAJOR BENEFITS

Bilberry extract is the leading herbal remedy for maintaining healthy vision and managing various eye disorders. In particular, bilberry helps the retina, the light-sensitive portion of the eye, adapt properly to both dark and light. It has been widely used to treat night blindness, as well as poor vision that can result from daytime glare.

With its ability to strengthen tiny blood vessels (capillaries)—and, in turn, facilitate the delivery of oxygen-rich blood to the eyes—bilberry may also play a significant role in preventing and treating degenerative diseases of the retina (retinopathy). In one study, 31 patients were treated with bilberry extract daily for four weeks. Use of the extract fortified the capillaries and reduced hemorrhaging in the eyes, especially in cases of diabetes-related retinopathy.

 ALERT

SIDE EFFECTS

- At therapeutic doses, bilberry appears to be very safe and has no known side effects, even when taken long term. However, it's a good idea to avoid taking more than 480 mg of bilberry a day.

CAUTION

- While the dried fruits of the bilberry plant are safe to use, it's probably best to refrain from ingesting the leaves because so little is known about their safety or effectiveness.

- **Reminder:** If you have a medical condition, talk to your doctor before taking supplements.

In addition, bilberry is useful for preventing macular degeneration (a progressive disorder affecting the central part of the retina) and cataracts (loss of transparency of the eye's lens)—two leading causes of vision loss in older people. A study of 50 patients with age-related cataracts found that bilberry extract combined with vitamin E supplements inhibited cataract formation in almost all of the participants.

Because it can strengthen collagen—the abundant protein that forms the "backbone" of healthy connective tissue—bilberry may also be valuable in preventing and treating glaucoma, a disease caused by excessive pressure within the eye.

ADDITIONAL BENEFITS

Because the anthocyanosides in bilberry improve blood flow in capillaries, as well as in larger blood vessels, bilberry in standardized extract form may be worthwhile for people with poor circulation in their extremities. It's helpful for varicose veins and for the pain and burning of hemorrhoids. People who bruise easily may also benefit from the salutary effect that bilberry has on capillaries.

Although more study is needed, limited data indicate that bilberry may have other uses as well. One study showed that long-term use of bilberry extract improved the vision of normally nearsighted people—although how it produced this effect is unknown.

Preliminary results in women show that bilberry helps treat menstrual cramps because anthocyanosides relax smooth muscle, including the uterus. And research studies done in animals suggest that bilberry anthocyanosides may fight stomach ulcers.

▼ HOW TO TAKE IT

DOSAGE
Normal dosages range from 40 mg to 160 mg of bilberry extract two or three times a day. The lower dose is generally recommended for long-term use, including prevention of macular degeneration; higher doses—up to 320 mg a day—may be needed to prevent retinal disease in diabetes.

GUIDELINES FOR USE
• Bilberry can be taken with or without food.

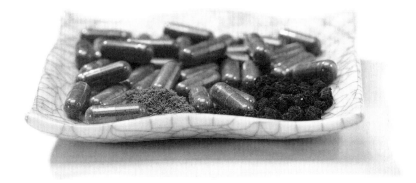

Bilberry, available in capsule form, is now a popular herbal remedy for treating a number of eye disorders.

SHOPPING HINTS

■ When buying bilberry, choose an extract standardized to contain 25% to 37% anthocyanosides, the active ingredients in the herb. (Actually, one particular type of anthocyanoside, called anthocyanidin, determines this standardized dose.) Standardized extracts help assure that you get the same amount of active compounds in each dose.

■ A convenient way to buy bilberry is in a "Vision" combination product., which may also include zinc, beta-carotene, vitamin A, lutein, and grape seed extract.

FACTS & TIPS

■ In Europe, bilberry is commonly recommended as part of conventional medical therapy, particularly for eye disorders. German doctors also prescribe bilberry tea for the relief of diarrhea. To make the tea, pour a cup of very hot water over 1 or 2 tablespoons of dried whole berries (or 2 or 3 teaspoons of crushed berries); steep for 10 minutes and strain. You can drink up to three cups of bilberry tea a day. The tea can also be cooled and used as a gargle to treat mouth and throat inflammations.

DID YOU KNOW?

Bilberry extracts contain between 100 and 250 times the amount of active ingredients (anthocyanosides) found in fresh bilberry fruit.

BIOTIN AND PANTOTHENIC ACID

It's surprising that these two members of the B-vitamin family don't get more attention. They work together at the most basic level to produce enzymes that trigger many bodily functions. In addition, biotin promotes healthy hair and nails, and pantothenic acid appears to play a valuable role in how the body deals with stress.

COMMON USES

Biotin

■ Promotes healthy nails and hair.

■ Helps the body use carbohydrates, fats, and protein.

■ May improve blood sugar control in people with diabetes.

Pantothenic acid

■ Promotes healthy function of the central nervous system.

■ Helps the body use carbohydrates, fats, and protein.

■ May improve symptoms of chronic fatigue syndrome, migraines, heartburn, and allergies.

FORMS

■ Capsule

■ Tablet

■ Softgel

■ Liquid

▼ WHAT IT IS

The names of these two vitamins suggest their widespread presence in the body. Both words have Greek roots: *pantothenic* from *pantos*, which means "everywhere," and *biotin* from *bios*, which means "life."

Because these vitamins are in many foods, deficiencies are virtually nonexistent. Biotin is also produced by intestinal bacteria, though this form may be difficult for the body to use.

Multivitamins and B-complex vitamins usually include biotin and pantothenic acid (also called vitamin B_5) and both are also available as individual supplements. The main form of biotin is d-biotin. Pantothenic acid comes in two forms: pantethine and calcium pantothenate; the latter is suitable for most purposes and is less expensive than pantethine.

▼ WHAT IT DOES

Both biotin and pantothenic acid are involved in the breakdown of carbohydrates, fats, and protein from foods and in the production of enzymes. Biotin plays a special role in helping the body use glucose, its basic fuel, and it also promotes healthy nails and hair. The body needs pantothenic acid to maintain proper communication between the brain and nervous system and to produce certain stress hormones.

MAJOR BENEFITS

Biotin improves the quality of weak and brittle fingernails and may help slow hair loss, if it's caused by a biotin deficiency. Research suggests the overproduction of stress hormones during long periods of emotional upset, depression, or anxiety increases the need for pantothenic acid, which is used to manufacture these hormones.

Because stress is a factor in quitting smoking, migraines, and chronic fatigue, pantothenic acid may be useful for these conditions. In combination with the B vitamins choline and thiamin, pantothenic acid can be an effective heartburn remedy; it also helps reduce nasal congestion of allergies.

ADDITIONAL BENEFITS

In high doses, biotin may help people with diabetes, increasing the body's response to insulin so blood sugar (glucose) levels stay low. In addition,

---

 ALERT

SIDE EFFECTS

• Diarrhea can result from taking 10 grams (10,000 mg) or more a day of pantothenic acid.

CAUTION

• Very high doses of biotin (more than 8 mg a day) used to treat diabetes may alter insulin requirements.

• **Reminder:** If you have a medical condition, talk to your doctor before taking supplements.

it may protect against the nerve damage that sometimes occurs in diabetes (called diabetic neuropathy).

▼ HOW MUCH YOU NEED

There is no RDA for biotin or pantothenic acid, but an an Adequate Intake (AI) has been established. For biotin it is 30 mcg and for pantothenic acid 5 mg a day for both men and women. These amounts appear to be enough to maintain normal body functioning, but for treating specific diseases or disorders, higher doses may be needed.

IF YOU GET TOO LITTLE
Deficiencies of biotin or pantothenic acid are virtually unknown in adults. Long-term use of antibiotics or anti-seizure medications, however, can lead to less-than-optimal levels of biotin.

IF YOU GET TOO MUCH
There are no known serious adverse effects from high doses of biotin or pantothenic acid. Some people report diarrhea when taking doses of 10 grams a day or more of pantothenic acid.

▼ HOW TO TAKE IT

DOSAGE
For hair and nails: Take 1,000 to 1,200 mcg of biotin a day.
To aid in quitting smoking: Take 500 mg pantothenic acid twice a day.
During periods of stress: Take 100 mg of pantothenic acid a day as part of a vitamin B complex.
For migraines: Take 400 mg of pantothenic acid twice a day.

For chronic fatigue syndrome: Take 500 mg of pantothenic acid twice a day.
For chronic heartburn: Take 1,000 mg of pantothenic acid twice a day along with 500 mg of thiamin first thing in the morning and 500 mg choline three times a day.
For allergies: Take 500 mg of pantothenic acid three times a day.
For diabetes: Talk with your doctor about taking high doses of biotin to help or even prevent diabetic neuropathy.

GUIDELINES FOR USE
• Most people will get enough biotin and pantothenic acid from a daily multivitamin or a B-complex supplement. Individual supplements are necessary only to treat a specific disorder.

• In most cases, take individual supplements with meals.

▼ OTHER SOURCES

Biotin is found in liver, soy products, nuts, oatmeal, rice, barley, legumes, cauliflower, and whole wheat. Organ meats, fish, poultry, whole grains, yogurt, and legumes are the best sources of pantothenic acid.

FACTS & TIPS
■ If you eat a lot of processed foods, you should consider taking a supplement with pantothenic acid, because this vitamin is easily destroyed in processing. Bread and cereal, for example, contain half the pantothenic acid found in the original whole grains. Even more pantothenic acid (70%) is lost when poultry or fish is frozen and thawed or when beans are canned (80%).

■ Biotin helps keep hair healthy, but—except in rare cases of biotin deficiency—it can't prevent baldness as some claim. Nor can pantothenic acid forestall the normal graying of hair that occurs with age.

LATEST FINDINGS
■ Biotin can increase the thickness of nails by an average of 25%, according to a study from Switzerland. Six months of taking biotin supplements improved brittle nails in two-thirds of the study's participants.

DID YOU KNOW?
You'd have to eat about 2½ cups of wheat germ to get 7 mg of pantothenic acid.

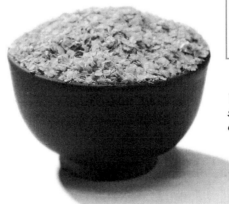

Wheat germ is a good food source of pantothenic acid, one of the B vitamins.

BLACK COHOSH *(Cimicifuga racemosa)*

Though baby boomers may claim black cohosh as the new "in" herb, its healing abilities were clearly recognized more than a century ago, when Native American and pioneer women singled out the root of this plant as one of the most useful natural medicines for treating menstrual and menopausal complaints.

COMMON USES

■ Reduces menopausal symptoms, particularly hot flashes.

■ Eases menstrual pain and other difficulties, such as PMS.

■ Works as an anti-inflammatory; relieves muscle pain.

■ Helps clear mucous membranes and relieve coughs.

FORMS

■ Capsule

■ Tablet

■ Tincture

■ Dried herb/Tea

▼ WHAT IT IS

Long used to treat "women's problems," black cohosh ("black" describes the dark color of the root; "cohosh" is derived from an Algonquian word for "rough") grows up to eight feet high and is distinguished by its tall stalks of fluffy white flowers. This member of the buttercup family is also known as bugbane, squawroot, rattle root, or *Cimicifuga racemosa,* its botanical name.

This herb's most common nickname, black snakeroot, describes its gnarled root, the part of the plant that is used medicinally. Contained in the root is a complex network of natural chemicals, some of them as powerful as the most modern pharmaceuticals.

▼ WHAT IT DOES

Traditionally, black cohosh has long been prescribed to treat menstrual problems, pain after childbirth, nervous disorders, and joint pain. Today, the herb is recommended primarily for relief of the hot flashes that some women experience during menopause.

MAJOR BENEFITS

In Europe and increasingly in the United States, black cohosh is a popular remedy for hot flashes, vaginal dryness, and other menopausal symptoms. Scientific study has shown that black cohosh can reduce levels of LH (luteinizing hormone), which is produced by the brain's pituitary gland. The rise in LH that occurs during menopause is thought to be one cause of hot flashes.

In addition, black cohosh contains phytoestrogens, plant compounds that have an effect similar to that of estrogen produced by the body. Phytoestrogens bind to hormone receptors in the breast, uterus, and elsewhere in the body, easing menopausal symptoms without increasing the risk of breast cancer, a possible side effect of hormone replacement therapy (HRT). In

 ALERT

SIDE EFFECTS
• Though it has virtually no toxic effects, black cohosh may cause stomach upset, slight weight gain, and dizziness in some women. It may also lower blood pressure.

• A very high dose can cause nausea, vomiting, reduced pulse rate, heavy perspiration, and headache. Consult your doctor immediately.

CAUTION
• Never use black cohosh while pregnant or breast-feeding.

• The herb's safety and effectiveness remain unclear for women with estrogen-sensitive cancers.

• This herb may interfere with hormonal medications (birth control pills or estrogen), so check with your doctor.

• Be careful if you're on a hypertension medication; black cohosh may intensify the drug's blood pressure-lowering effect.

• **Reminder:** If you have a medical condition, talk to your doctor before taking supplements.

fact, some experts think phytoestrogens may even help prevent breast cancer by keeping the body's own estrogen from locking onto breast cells.

ADDITIONAL BENEFITS

As a result of its antispasmodic properties, black cohosh can alleviate menstrual cramps by increasing blood flow to the uterus and reducing the intensity of uterine contractions. This action also makes it useful during labor and after childbirth. Because it evens out hormone levels, it may benefit women with premenstrual syndrome (PMS); however, the herb chasteberry is probably better for this condition.

Although these effects are less frequently noted, black cohosh has demonstrated some mildly sedating and anti-inflammatory capabilities, which may be particularly valuable in treating muscle aches, as well as in relieving nerve-related pain such as sciatica or neuralgia.

Because it has the ability to help clear mucus from the body, black cohosh has been recommended for coughs. This herb has also been shown to be effective as a treatment for ringing in the ears (tinnitus).

▼ HOW TO TAKE IT

DOSAGE

For menopausal or PMS symptoms: Take 20 mg of black cohosh twice a day or 40 mg once a day; for PMS, begin treatment a week to 10 days before your period.
For menstrual cramps: Take 40 mg three times a day as needed.

GUIDELINES FOR USE

• Black cohosh can be taken at any time of day, but to reduce the chance of stomach upset, you may prefer to use it with meals.

• Allow four to eight weeks to see its benefits. Many experts recommend a six-month limit on taking black cohosh, though recent studies show that longer use seems to be safe and free of significant side effects.

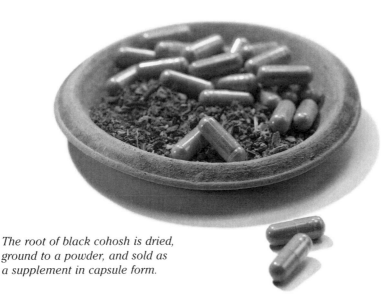

The root of black cohosh is dried, ground to a powder, and sold as a supplement in capsule form.

SHOPPING HINTS

■ Look for capsules or tablets containing extracts standardized to contain 2.5% of triterpene glycosides, the active components in black cohosh. Liquid forms should be standardized to 5% triterpenes.

FACTS & TIPS

■ Compresses soaked in a black cohosh tea can be used to soothe sore muscles and aching joints. Boil the dried root in water for 20 to 30 minutes. Let the liquid cool a bit (it should still be hot, but not hot enough to burn your skin). Then apply the warm compresses to the skin over the affected area for about 20 minutes.

■ Though some experts think that black cohosh helps reduce hot flashes and vaginal dryness as effectively as hormone replacement therapy (HRT), there's no evidence that this herb offers the protection against osteoporosis that HRT is believed to provide.

DID YOU KNOW?

Black cohosh was the main ingredient in one of the most popular folk medicines of all times—Lydia Pinkham's Vegetable Compound. Widely used in the early 1900s, this "women's tonic" is still available today. Ironically, the current formula no longer contains any of this helpful native herb.

CALCIUM

Renowned for preventing—or at least minimizing—the devastating effects of osteoporosis (age-related bone thinning), calcium is now also thought to lower high blood pressure and help prevent colon cancer. Because this important mineral is often seriously lacking in the modern American diet, supplements may be needed.

COMMON USES

- Maintains bones and teeth.
- Helps prevent progressive bone loss and osteoporosis.
- Aids heart and muscle contraction, nerve impulses, and blood clotting.
- May help lower blood pressure in people with hypertension.
- Eases heartburn.

FORMS

- Tablet
- Capsule
- Softgel
- Powder
- Liquid

▼ WHAT IT IS

Although it's the most abundant mineral in the body, most adults get just half the calcium they need each day. Eating enough calcium-rich foods may be difficult, but you can prevent a deficiency by taking supplements.

A wide array of products line store shelves. The most common forms are calcium carbonate, calcium citrate, calcium citrate malate, calcium gluconate, calcium phosphate, and calcium lactate. A supplement's elemental (or pure) calcium depends on its accompanying compound. Calcium carbonate (useful in antacids to relieve heartburn) provides 40% elemental calcium, while calcium gluconate supplies 9%.

The lower the calcium content, the more pills you need to meet recommended amounts. The amount of elemental calcium you absorb (and use) differs too; for most people, the elemental calcium in calcium citrate is absorbed best.

▼ WHAT IT DOES

The majority of the body's calcium is stored in the bones and teeth, where it provides strength and structure. The small amount circulating in the bloodstream helps move nutrients across cell membranes and plays a role in producing the hormones and enzymes that regulate digestion and metabolism. Calcium is also needed for normal communication among nerve cells, for blood clotting, for wound healing, and for muscle contraction.

To have enough of this mineral available in the blood to perform vital functions, the body will steal it from the bones. Over time, too many calcium withdrawals leave bones porous and fragile. Only an adequate daily calcium intake will maintain healthy levels in the blood—and provide enough extra for the bones to absorb as a reserve.

PREVENTION

Getting enough calcium throughout life is a central factor in preventing osteoporosis, the bone-thinning disease that leads to a higher risk of hip and vertebrae fractures, spinal deformities, and loss of height. The body is best equipped to absorb calcium and build up bone mass before age 35, but it's never too late to increase your intake

ALERT

CAUTION

- People who have thyroid or kidney disease should check with their doctor before taking calcium.

- Calcium may interact with certain drugs. It can decrease the absorption of tetracycline antibiotics, and taken with thiazide diuretics, it can increase calcium to dangerous levels.

- **Reminder:** If you have a medical condition, talk to your doctor before taking supplements.

of it. Several studies show that even in people over age 65, taking calcium supplements and eating calcium-rich foods help maintain bone density and reduce the risk of fractures.

ADDITIONAL BENEFITS
By limiting the irritating effects of bile acids in the colon, calcium may reduce the incidence of colon cancer. Other research indicates that diets including plenty of calcium—as well as fruits and vegetables—may actually help lower blood pressure as much as some prescription medications do.

▼ HOW MUCH YOU NEED

Official dietary guidelines, now called Adequate Intake (AI) levels, were recently increased to reflect new findings about the body's daily calcium needs. The AI is currently 1,000 mg for men and women ages 19 to 50, and 1,200 mg for ages 51 to 70 and older.

IF YOU GET TOO LITTLE
A prolonged calcium deficiency can lead to bone abnormalities, such as osteoporosis. Muscle spasms can result from low levels of calcium in the blood.

IF YOU GET TOO MUCH
A daily calcium intake as high as 2,500 mg from a combination of food and supplements appears to be safe. However, taking calcium supplements may impair the body's absorption of the minerals zinc, iron, and magnesium.

And very high doses of calcium from supplements might lead to kidney stones. Calcium carbonate may cause gas or constipation; if this becomes a problem, switch to calcium citrate.

▼ HOW TO TAKE IT

DOSAGE
Be sure to get the recommended amount of 1,000 to 1,200 mg of elemental calcium a day from foods, supplements, or both. It's often a good idea to also add supplemental magnesium when taking calcium.

GUIDELINES FOR USE
• To enhance absorption, divide your supplement dose so that you don't consume more than 600 mg of calcium at any one time.

• Be sure to take the supplements with food.

▼ OTHER SOURCES

The most familiar and plentiful sources of calcium are dairy products, such as milk, yogurt, or cheese. Choose low- or nonfat varieties: They're better for you and also contain slightly more calcium, ounce for ounce.

Orange juice fortified with calcium malate, canned salmon and sardines (eaten with the soft bones), collard greens, arugula, broccoli, and almonds are good nondairy sources.

SHOPPING HINTS

■ If you are over age 65, try to purchase calcium citrate. People over this age often lack sufficient stomach acid to absorb calcium carbonate effectively.

FACTS & TIPS

■ Avoid calcium supplements made from dolomite, oyster shells, or bonemeal because such compounds may contain unacceptable levels of lead.

■ Calcium cannot be absorbed without vitamin D, which is made by the skin in response to sunlight. Because your body's ability to convert sunlight to vitamin D declines with age, your safest bet is to get 200 to 400 IU of vitamin D a day in your diet (fortified milk is the best source) or in supplement form. You can also buy calcium supplements with vitamin D.

■ Spinach is not a good source of calcium. It contains high levels of substances called oxalates, which lock up the calcium and limit the amount available to the body. The oxalates don't interfere with calcium absorption from other foods eaten at the same time, however.

DID YOU KNOW?

You'd have to eat nearly 80 florets of broccoli to get the 1,200 mg of calcium recommended daily.

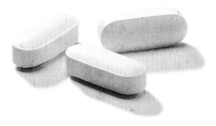

CAROTENOIDS

The built-in pigments that give some fruits and vegetables their rich red, orange, and yellow colors are called carotenoids. Scientists are now discovering that these natural compounds are also potent disease fighters. If your diet doesn't contain enough of them, nutritional supplements can be a handy option.

COMMON USES

- May lower the risk of certain types of cancers, including prostate and lung cancer.
- May provide protection against heart disease.
- Slow the development of age-related macular degeneration.
- Enhance immunity.

FORMS

- Capsule
- Tablet
- Softgel

▼ WHAT IT IS

Although more than 600 carotenoid pigments have been identified in foods, it appears that only six of them are used in significant ways by the blood or tissues of the body. Besides beta-carotene (see page 34), which is probably the best-known carotenoid, these substances include alpha-carotene, lycopene, lutein, zeaxanthin, and cryptoxanthin.

Though carotenoids are found in various fruits and vegetables, the foods that represent the most concentrated sources may not be part of your daily fare. Alpha-carotene is found in carrots and pumpkin; lycopene is abundant in red fruits, such as watermelon, red grapefruit, guava, and especially processed tomatoes. Lutein and zeaxanthin are plentiful in dark green vegetables, pumpkin, and red peppers; and cryptoxanthin is present in mangoes, oranges, and peaches.

To prevent certain diseases, supplements providing a mix of the six key carotenoids may be in order.

▼ WHAT IT DOES

The primary benefit of carotenoids lies in their antioxidant potential. Antioxidants are compounds that in the body neutralize disease-causing unstable oxygen molecules called free radicals. Though the carotenoids are similar, each acts on a specific type of body tissue. In addition, alpha-carotene and cryptoxanthin can be converted into vitamin A in the body, but not to the same extent as beta-carotene.

PREVENTION

Carotenoids may guard against certain types of cancer, apparently by limiting the abnormal growth of cells. Lycopene, for instance, appears to inhibit prostate cancer formation. Researchers at Harvard University found men who ate 10 or more servings a week of tomato-based foods—tomatoes are the richest dietary source of lycopene—cut their risk of prostate cancer by nearly 45%. Lycopene may also be effective against some cancers of the stomach and digestive tract.

Studies show that high intakes of alpha-carotene, lutein, and zeaxanthin

 ALERT

SIDE EFFECTS
- Large doses of carotenoids (through food or supplements) can turn your skin orange, especially the palms of your hands and the soles of your feet. This effect is harmless and will gradually go away if you reduce your intake of these pigments.

- Taking high doses of individual carotenoids may interfere with the workings of other carotenoids in your body and could even cause harm.

CAUTION
- **Reminder:** If you have a medical condition, talk to your doctor before taking supplements.

decrease the risk of lung cancer, and that cryptoxanthin and alpha-carotene lower the risk of cervical cancer.

In addition, carotenoids may fight heart disease. In a survey of 1,300 elderly people, the ones who ate the most carotenoid-rich foods had half the risk of developing heart disease and a 75% lower chance of heart attack than did those who ate the least amount of these foods. This was true even after researchers adjusted for other heart-disease risk factors, such as smoking and high cholesterol levels.

Scientists believe that all carotenoids, and particularly alpha-carotene and lycopene, block the formation of LDL ("bad") cholesterol. High LDL levels can lead to heart attacks and other cardiovascular problems.

ADDITIONAL BENEFITS
The carotenoids lutein and zeaxanthin promote clear vision by absorbing the sun's harmful ultraviolet rays and neutralizing free radicals in the retina (the light-sensitive portion of the eye). This may help reduce the risk of macular degeneration, an age-related vision disorder that is the leading cause of blindness in older adults. Other carotenoids may prevent damage to the lens of the eye and so decrease the risk of cataracts.

Preliminary studies now also indicate there may be a link between low levels of carotenoids and various menstrual disorders. In addition, other studies show that, even after the onset of cancer, a diet that is high in carotenoids may improve the overall prognosis of the disease.

▼ HOW TO TAKE IT

DOSAGE
If you don't eat a wide variety of carotenoid-rich foods, take a supplement that contains mixed carotenoids—alpha-carotene, beta-carotene, lycopene, lutein, zeaxanthin, and cryptoxanthin—and supplies a minimum of 25,000 IU vitamin A activity each day. Higher doses of mixed carotenoids may be recommended for the prevention of specific disorders.

GUIDELINES FOR USE
• Take carotenoid supplements with foods that contain a bit of fat, which helps the body absorb the carotenoids more effectively.

• Some experts also believe that your body will absorb more of these nutrients if you divide the total daily amount of carotenoids you plan to take in half and have them at two different times during the day.

FACTS & TIPS
■ Women who take oral contraceptives and postmenopausal women who use estrogen-based hormone replacement therapy (HRT) have reduced levels of carotenoids in their blood. A mixed carotenoid supplement can be worthwhile for women in both of these groups.

■ Cooked tomatoes contain less water and consequently more lycopene than raw ones. And some experts think that the oil used in tomato sauce makes the lycopene more absorbable.

LATEST FINDINGS
■ In a major European study, lycopene was shown to help prevent heart attacks. Men who consumed large amounts of lycopene had only half the risk of a heart attack of men who consumed small amounts. Lycopene's protective effect was most beneficial to nonsmokers.

DID YOU KNOW?
Dark green vegetables contain carotenoids. The green chlorophyll masks the yellow-orange pigments that they contain.

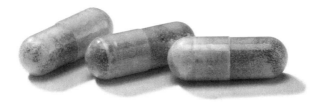

Although capsules for individual carotenoids such as lycopene (left) are available, it's best to take a mixed carotenoid supplement.

CAT'S CLAW *(Uncaria tomentosa, U. guianensis)*

Although Western researchers have studied cat's claw since the 1970s and European doctors have used it since the 1980s, popular interest in this herb has surged only recently. Studies suggest it may give the immune system a needed boost, which may be particularly beneficial for people who are fighting cancer.

COMMON USES

- May enhance immunity, making it useful for sinusitis and other infections.
- Supports cancer treatment.
- May help relieve chronic pain.
- Reduces pain and inflammation from gout or arthritis.

FORMS

- Tablet
- Capsule
- Softgel
- Liquid extract/Tincture
- Dried herb/Tea

▼ WHAT IT IS

In the Amazon basin, one woody tropical vine twining up trees in the rain forest features at the base of its leaves two curved thorns that resemble the claws of a cat. The herb derived from the inner bark or roots of this plant is known as cat's claw, or *uña de gato* (its Spanish name).

Although there are dozens of related species, two specific ones, *Uncaria tomentosa* and *U. guianensis,* are harvested in the wild (primarily in Peru and Brazil) for medicinal purposes. Large pieces of their bark are a common sight in South American farmers' markets; native Indians have long made tea from the bark and used it to treat wounds, stomach ills, arthritis, cancer, and other ailments.

▼ WHAT IT DOES

Modern scientific studies have identified several active ingredients in cat's claw that enhance the activity of the immune system and inhibit inflammation. Their presence may help explain why this herb traditionally has been employed to fight cancer, arthritis, dysentery, ulcers, and other infectious and inflammatory conditions.

MAJOR BENEFITS

In Germany and Austria, physicians prescribe cat's claw to stimulate the immune response in cancer patients, many of whom may be weakened by chemotherapy, radiation, or other conventional cancer treatments.

Several compounds in cat's claw—some of which have been studied for decades—may account for its cancer-fighting and immune-boosting effects. In the 1970s, researchers reported that the inner bark and root contain compounds called procyanidolic oligomers (PCOs), which inhibit tumors in animals. In the 1980s, German scientists identified other compounds in cat's claw that enhance the immune system, in part by stimulating immune cells called phagocytes that engulf and devour viruses, bacteria, and other disease-causing microorganisms.

Then, in 1993, an Italian study detected another class of compounds, called quinovic acid glycosides, that have

ALERT

SIDE EFFECTS

- There have been few studies on the safety of this plant. Side effects may include low blood pressure and unusual bleeding and bruising; discontinue use and consult a doctor if such reactions occur.

CAUTION

- Never take cat's claw if you are pregnant, considering pregnancy, or breast-feeding. Its safety is not established in these situations, and the herb has been associated with excessive bleeding.

- **Reminder:** If you have a medical condition, talk to your doctor before taking supplements.

multiple benefits. These act as antioxidants, ridding the body of cell-damaging molecules called free radicals. They also kill viruses, reduce inflammation, and inhibit the transformation of normal cells into cancerous ones.

In addition to its anti-tumor potential, cat's claw may be of value in combating stubborn infections such as sinusitis.

ADDITIONAL BENEFITS

Traditionally the herb has been relied on to treat pain. Because of its anti-inflammatory properties, it may be effective in relieving joint pain caused by arthritis or gout. Additional studies are needed, however, to define the precise role that cat's claw plays in treating arthritis as well as other inflammatory complaints.

Some preliminary reports found that cat's claw, in conjunction with conventional AIDS drugs, may benefit people infected with HIV, because it seems to boost the immune response; further studies are necessary, however.

Some experts caution against taking the herb for chronic conditions affecting the immune system, including tuberculosis, multiple sclerosis, and rheumatoid arthritis, because they believe it may overstimulate the immune system and make symptoms worse. Other doctors, however, recommend it for autoimmune disorders, including rheumatoid arthritis and lupus. More research is needed.

▼ HOW TO TAKE IT

DOSAGE

Take 250 mg of a standardized extract in pill form twice a day. Alternatively, consume 1 to 2 ml (about 30 drops) of the liquid extract three times a day in a glass of water. Or use as directed by a health-care practitioner.

Pills containing the crude herb (the ground root or inner bark in a nonconcentrated form) are often available in 500 or 1,000 mg capsules. Have these twice daily (up to 2,000 mg a day).

Cat's claw tea is sold in health-food stores; use 1 or 2 teaspoons of dried herb per cup of very hot water (follow package directions). You can drink up to three cups a day.

GUIDELINES FOR USE

• You can combine or rotate cat's claw with other immune-stimulating herbs, such as echinacea, goldenseal, reishi and maitake mushrooms, astragalus, or pau d'arco.

• Pregnant or breast-feeding women should avoid cat's claw. In Peru, cat's claw has been long valued as a contraceptive; in animals, it stimulates uterine contractions. This effect suggests the herb could induce a miscarriage.

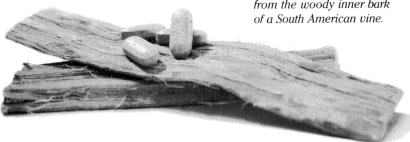

Cat's claw tablets are made from the woody inner bark of a South American vine.

SHOPPING HINTS

■ Whenever possible, select standardized extracts of cat's claw to help guarantee that you're getting a proper dose of the herb. Look for preparations that are standardized to contain 3% alkaloids and 15% polyphenols.

■ Buy supplements made from *Uncaria tomentosa* or *U. guianensis*. Many products on the market do not actually include cat's claw, but are herbs that look like or carry the same name as the real thing. These include preparations from the southwestern United States containing a completely unrelated plant (*Acacia greggii*) that's also called cat's claw. A month's supply of true cat's claw from a reputable supplier will likely cost $20 to $30.

FACTS & TIPS

■ Even though cat's claw root may contain higher percentages of active ingredients than its inner bark, the latter is preferred for ecological reasons. When the inner bark is harvested, it is possible to keep the tree alive, whereas uprooting the plant will endanger it. If you purchase a standardized extract made from inner bark, you'll get a guaranteed level of active ingredients.

DID YOU KNOW?

In Germany and Austria, cat's claw extract is considered a potent medicine and is typically dispensed only with a doctor's prescription.

CAYENNE *(Capsicum species)*

This fiery spice, made from dried hot peppers, is said to have originated in Cayenne, French Guiana. Ever since a physician sailing with Columbus first described this pungent fruit, the cayenne pepper's popularity has grown. Today it's valued as a topical painkiller (especially for arthritic joints), digestive aid, and food enhancer.

COMMON USES

Topical cream and ointment

■ Relieve arthritis pain.

■ Reduce nerve pain of shingles (post-herpetic neuralgia), diabetes, surgery, or trigeminal neuralgia (tic douloureux).

Tablet, capsule, and tincture

■ Alleviate indigestion.

FORMS

■ Cream/Ointment

■ Tablet

■ Capsule

■ Softgel

■ Tincture/Liquid

■ Fresh or dried herb

▼ WHAT IT IS

Derived from several varieties of the *Capsicum* species, cayenne is a hot pepper famous for the fiery taste it brings to Cajun, Mexican, Indian, Asian, and other cuisines. It's a cousin of the bell peppers used in salads and the hot peppers that produce chili powder and hot sauces, but it's unrelated to common black table pepper.

The main active ingredient in cayenne—and what gives the pepper its hotness—is capsaicin (pronounced cap-SAY-sin), an irritating, oily chemical that's also the prime component of pepper sprays sold for self-defense.

▼ WHAT IT DOES

When applied to the skin, capsaicin is an effective painkiller. It causes the depletion of a component in nerve cells called substance P, which transmits pain impulses to the brain. When ingested in supplement form or in food, cayenne is believed to aid digestion.

MAJOR BENEFITS

Regular application to the skin of a cream or ointment containing capsaicin can be very effective for relieving the pain of arthritis. It also helps ease lingering post-shingles pain, as well as painful nerve damage from diabetes and from surgery (such as a mastectomy or an amputation).

Preliminary studies indicate cayenne cream may have other beneficial uses. It may reduce the itching of psoriasis (the itching sensation follows the same nerve pathways as pain). The cream has also shown promise in relieving the aches and pains of fibromyalgia and the coldness in the extremities caused by Raynaud's disease.

ADDITIONAL BENEFITS

Fresh peppers, tinctures, teas, tablets, and capsules are said to stimulate digestion and help relieve gas and ulcers by increasing blood circulation in the stomach and bowel and by promoting the secretion of natural digestive juices.

ALERT

SIDE EFFECTS

• Cayenne cream or ointment frequently generates warmth or a mildly unpleasant burning sensation that lasts half an hour or so during the first few days of topical application, but this effect usually disappears after several days of regular use.

• Taken internally, cayenne may cause stomach pain or diarrhea. Capsaicin in the stool can produce a burning sensation during bowel movements.

• Cayenne can sometimes trigger coughing, sneezing, tearing, or an irritated throat. These may be a result of using too much cream or inhaling the powder.

CAUTION

• Never apply cayenne cream to raw or open skin. And avoid touching your eyes and contact lenses: The burning sensation can be intense.

• **Reminder:** If you have a medical condition, talk to your doctor before taking supplements.

Liquid forms mixed with water can be used as a gargle to soothe a sore throat. Special nasal preparations have been studied that may relieve congestion, fight colds, and alleviate the piercing pain of cluster headaches (try these only under a doctor's supervision).

Claims that cayenne may reduce heart disease risk (by lowering blood cholesterol and triglyceride levels) or help prevent cancer (by providing vitamin C and other antioxidants) are unfounded.

▼ HOW TO TAKE IT

DOSAGE

For external use: Cayenne cream or ointment containing 0.025% to 0.075% capsaicin is most effective with regular, daily use; apply it thinly over the affected areas at least three or four times a day for pain, rubbing it in well. Pain may take several weeks to subside. *For internal use:* Follow the package instructions.

GUIDELINES FOR USE

For external use

• Because sensitivity to cayenne varies, test it first on a small, particularly painful area. If it works—and this may take a week or more—and causes no lasting discomfort, you can enlarge the coverage area.

• To avoid getting cayenne in the eyes, wash your hands after use with warm, soapy water or wear latex gloves during application and promptly discard them; you can also cover the area with a loose bandage.

• If cayenne does get in your eyes (or other moist mucous membranes) it may cause intense pain and burning, but no lasting damage. Flush the affected area with water or milk. To remove cayenne from the skin, wash the area with warm, soapy water. Vinegar may also work, but don't use it in or near your eyes.

• If you're using cayenne cream to relieve pain in the fingers or hands, wait 30 minutes before washing it off to allow the cream to penetrate the skin. In the meantime, avoid touching contact lenses and sensitive areas, such as your eyes and nose.

• Store cayenne cream away from light and extreme heat or cold, and keep it out of the reach of children.

For internal use:

• Cayenne can be taken with or without food. No adverse effects have been reported in pregnant or breast-feeding women who use it internally or externally, but discontinue it if a nursing baby becomes irritable.

Cayenne peppers are the source of digestion-aiding capsules and painkilling skin creams.

SHOPPING HINTS

■ Doctors frequently write prescriptions for cayenne (capsaicin) creams. But many nonprescription hot pepper creams at the same potencies (0.025% to 0.075%) are available in drugstores and health-food stores. An over-the-counter cream might save you money.

■ To keep your feet warm, some herbal cayenne products are made to be sprinkled into socks. Although this remedy may be moderately effective, be careful when using such a product with young children, who could get cayenne in their eyes when they're changing their socks.

FACTS & TIPS

■ Cayenne can be used safely with NSAIDs (nonsteroidal anti-inflammatory drugs) and other arthritis medications. Such a combination may allow you to cut back on your medication dosage, reducing the likelihood of side effects. Check with your doctor before changing your dosage.

■ Hot peppers are measured in Scoville units (SU). Cayenne peppers ring in at 30,000 to 50,000 SU, jalapeño peppers at just 2,500 to 5,000 SU, and New Mexico hot peppers at 500 to 1,000 SU.

DID YOU KNOW?

Fresh or dried, cayenne peppers contain about 1.5% capsaicin—the painkilling ingredient that provides them with their legendary hotness.

CHAMOMILE (*Matricaria recutita*)

Sometimes called the world's most soothing plant, chamomile has traditionally been enjoyed as a tea that helps relax the nerves and ease a variety of digestive complaints. In concentrated form, this herb is increasingly found in pills, tinctures, and liquid extracts; it's also included in skin formulas to treat sores and rashes.

COMMON USES

- Promotes general relaxation and relieves anxiety.
- Alleviates insomnia.
- Heals mouth sores and treats diseases of the gums.
- Soothes skin rashes and burns, including sunburn.
- Relieves red and irritated eyes.
- Eases menstrual cramps.
- Treats bowel inflammation, digestive upset, and heartburn.

FORMS

- Capsule
- Dried herb/Tea
- Liquid extract/Tincture
- Oil
- Cream/Ointment

▼ WHAT IT IS

Chamomile is actually two herbs: German chamomile and Roman chamomile. The more popular (and the one discussed in this book) is German—sometimes called Hungarian—chamomile. It comes from the dried flowers of the *Matricaria recutita* plant (its older botanical names are *Matricaria chamomilla* and *Chamomilla recutita*).

The other type of chamomile, known variously as Roman or English chamomile (*Chamaemelum nobile* or *Anthemis nobilis*), has properties similar to those of the German species; it is sold mainly in Europe.

This herb has long been used to prepare a gently soothing tea. Because of its pleasing, applelike aroma and flavor (the name "chamomile" is derived from the Greek *kamai melon*, which means "ground apple"), many people find the ritual of brewing and sipping the tea a relaxing experience.

Concentrated chamomile extracts are also added to creams and lotions or packaged as pills or tinctures. The healing properties of the herb are related in part to its volatile oils, which contain a compound called apigenin as well as other therapeutic substances.

▼ WHAT IT DOES

Chamomile is a great soother. Its anti-inflammatory, antispasmodic, and infection-fighting effects can benefit the whole body—inside and out. When taken internally, it calms digestive upsets, relieves cramping, and relaxes the nerves. It also works externally on the skin and the mucous membranes of the mouth and eyes, relieving rashes, sores, and inflammation.

MAJOR BENEFITS

When Peter Rabbit's mother put him to bed, she gave him a spoonful of warm chamomile tea. Scientists have confirmed her wisdom. Studies in animals have shown chamomile contains substances that act on the same parts of the brain and nervous system that anti-anxiety drugs affect, promoting relaxation and reducing stress.

Chamomile appears to have a mildly sedating effect, but more important,

ALERT

SIDE EFFECTS

- Whether chamomile is used internally or externally, side effects are rare. Those taking higher-than-recommended doses of the herb have reported instances of nausea and vomiting.

- Though some red flags have been raised about possible allergic reactions, which cause bronchial tightness or skin rashes, these appear to be so rare that most people needn't worry about them.

CAUTION

- **Reminder:** If you have a medical condition, talk to your doctor before taking supplements.

it also calms the body, making it easier for the person who's taking it to fall asleep naturally.

In addition, the herb has a relaxing, anti-inflammatory effect on the smooth muscles that line the digestive tract: It helps ease a wide range of gastrointestinal complaints, including heartburn, diverticular disorders, and inflammatory bowel disease. In addition, its muscle-relaxing action may assist women who are suffering from menstrual cramps.

ADDITIONAL BENEFITS
Used externally, chamomile helps soothe skin inflammation. It contains bacteria-fighting compounds that may speed the healing of infections as well. A dressing soaked in chamomile tea, for instance, is often beneficial when applied to mild burns.

For sunburn, chamomile oil can be added to a cool bath or mixed with almond oil and rubbed on sunburned areas. Chamomile creams, available ready-made in health-food stores, may relieve sunburn, as well as skin rashes such as eczema.

The herb can also treat inflammation or infection of the eyes or mouth. Eyewashes made from the cooled tea may ease the redness or irritation of conjunctivitis and other eye inflammations; prepare a fresh batch of tea daily and store it in a sterile container. Used daily as a gargle or mouthwash, the tea can help heal mouth sores and prevent gum disease.

▼ HOW TO TAKE IT

DOSAGE
To make a soothing cup of chamomile tea: Pour a cup of very hot (not boiling) water over 2 teaspoons of dried flowers. Steep for five minutes and strain. Drink up to three cups a day or a cup at bedtime. The tea should be cooled thoroughly and kept sterile if you're using it on the skin or eyes. For the skin, add a few drops of chamomile oil to half an ounce of almond oil (or another neutral oil) or buy a ready-made cream.

Pills and liquids are also available; follow package directions. A single pill, or 1 to 2 teaspoons of liquid extract in water, has the therapeutic effects of a cup of tea.

GUIDELINES FOR USE
• Chamomile is gentle and can be used long term. It can be combined safely with prescription and over-the-counter drugs, as well as with other herbs and nutritional supplements.

• At recommended doses, the herb seems to be safe for children and pregnant and nursing women.

SHOPPING HINTS
■ Pills and liquid forms are formulated with concentrated extracts of chamomile. Look for standardized extracts that contain at least 1% apigenin, one of the herb's healing ingredients.

■ Check the labels of chamomile skin products carefully. Some feature the herb but contain only minuscule amounts. Buy creams or ointments that have at least 3% chamomile.

FACTS & TIPS
■ A chamomile bath can be very relaxing—and provide relief for dry, irritated skin or sunburn. Add 10 drops of chamomile oil, or several cups of chamomile tea, to a cool bath and soak for half an hour or longer.

■ To treat burns, stick with chamomile creams or teas rather than greasy ointments. The latter contain oils that can trap the heat, slow healing, and increase the risk of infection. Creams, on the other hand, are usually made with a non-oily base.

DID YOU KNOW?
Some people have successfully grown chamomile in their garden by simply tearing open a bag of chamomile tea and sprinkling its contents on the soil.

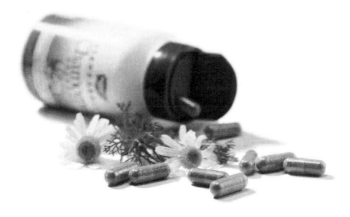

CHASTEBERRY *(Vitex agnus-castus)*

Although chasteberry has been used since ancient times for menstrual complaints, European doctors began prescribing it only in the 1950s. Today, it has become one of the most frequently recommended herbs in Europe for treating bloating, breast tenderness, and other common symptoms of premenstrual syndrome (PMS).

COMMON USES

■ Alleviates symptoms of premenstrual syndrome (PMS).

■ Regulates menstruation.

■ Promotes fertility.

■ Eases menopausal hot flashes.

FORMS

■ Liquid extract/Tincture

■ Tablet

■ Capsule

■ Dried herb/Tea

▼ WHAT IT IS

Also called vitex, chaste tree berry, or monk's pepper, chasteberry is the fruit of the chaste tree. Actually a small shrub with violet flower spikes and long, slender leaves, the chaste tree is native to the Mediterranean region, but grows in subtropical climates throughout the world. Its red berries are harvested in the fall and then dried. They resemble peppercorns in shape, and the taste they impart to a therapeutic cup of tea is distinctively peppery.

▼ WHAT IT DOES

The use of chasteberry for "female complaints" dates back to the time of Hippocrates. Although the herb does not actually contain hormones or hormonelike substances, it does spark the pituitary gland (located at the base of the brain) to send a signal to the ovaries to increase production of the female hormone progesterone.

Chasteberry also inhibits the excessive production of prolactin, a hormone that primarily regulates breast-milk production but has other less-understood actions as well.

MAJOR BENEFITS

Some scientists believe that women who routinely suffer from premenstrual syndrome (PMS) produce too little progesterone in the last two weeks of their menstrual cycle. This deficiency causes an imbalance in the body's natural estrogen-progesterone ratio. Chasteberry helps restore hormonal equilibrium, relieving such PMS-related complaints as irritability, bloating, and depression. Studies in Germany indicate that the herb offers at least some relief for PMS symptoms in about 90% of women—and in one-third of them, the symptoms disappear.

Chasteberry's prolactin-lowering action aids in reducing the breast pain and tenderness some women experience prior to menstruation, even if they have no other premenstrual symptoms.

ADDITIONAL BENEFITS

Because high levels of prolactin and low levels of progesterone in the body

---

 ALERT

SIDE EFFECTS

• Most people will not have any serious side effects from chasteberry.

• In a small percentage of women, studies have shown that stomach irritation or an itchy rash can occur. Discontinue using this herb if you develop any rash.

• Some women may experience an increased menstrual flow after taking chasteberry.

CAUTION

• Chasteberry affects hormone production, so it should not be used by women taking hormonal medications, including birth control pills and estrogen, or by those who are pregnant.

• **Reminder:** If you have a medical condition, talk to your doctor before taking supplements.

can inhibit monthly ovulation, chasteberry may be useful to those who are having trouble getting pregnant. The herb works best in women with mild or moderately low progesterone levels. When too much prolactin causes menstruation to stop (a condition called amenorrhea), the herb can help restore a normal monthly cycle.

Menopausal hot flashes are also the result of hormonal changes controlled by the pituitary gland, so women going through menopause may want to try chasteberry. Used either alone or in combination with other herbs such as dong quai or black cohosh, it can alleviate the periodic flushing and sweating that occur. Chasteberry is sometimes also recommended for menstrual-related acne.

▼ HOW TO TAKE IT

DOSAGE
Whether you're using chasteberry to treat infertility or to relieve PMS, breast tenderness, amenorrhea, or other menstrual disorders, the dose is the same.

In powdered extract form as a tablet or capsule: Take 225 mg standardized extract twice a day.
In liquid extract form: Add 30 drops to a glass of water and take three times a day.
For menopausal hot flashes: Take the same dosages as above (30 drops or 225 mg) twice a day.

GUIDELINES FOR USE
• Take chasteberry on an empty stomach to increase absorption; your first dose of the day should always be taken in the morning.

• Even after just 10 days, a woman with PMS symptoms will probably notice at least some improvement during her next menstrual cycle. However, it may take three months of use to benefit from the full effect of this herb. Six months of treatment with chasteberry may be necessary to correct infertility or amenorrhea.

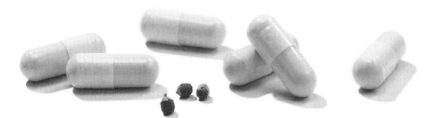

The tiny dark red fruit of the chasteberry tree contains the herb's active ingredients.

SHOPPING HINTS

■ Pill and liquid forms of chasteberry are formulated with the dried fruit of the plant. Look for standardized extracts that contain 0.5% agnusides, the active component of chasteberry.

■ Chasteberry is often included in combination "female" formulas, along with such other herbs as dong quai and black cohosh. Check the label to be sure you're getting enough of each herb for the supplement to be effective.

FACTS & TIPS

■ It may be difficult for you to take chasteberry tincture on an empty stomach, because the alcohol base of the solution can cause stomach irritation. Instead, try dividing the dose and taking half twice a day, after breakfast and lunch. Or switch to a pill form.

DID YOU KNOW?

Chasteberry is so named because it was believed to suppress the libido. In the Middle Ages, monks chewed on the dried berries to help them maintain their vows of celibacy. But in the amounts now recommended for treating PMS or other menstrual problems, chasteberry does not seem to dampen sexual desire.

CHROMIUM

The second best-selling mineral supplement after calcium in the United States, chromium has been hyped as a fat burner, muscle builder, treatment for diabetes, and weapon against heart disease. Though research shows that this mineral is essential for growth and health, its more spectacular claims remain controversial.

COMMON USES

- Essential for the breakdown of protein, fat, and carbohydrates.
- Helps the body maintain normal blood sugar (glucose) levels.
- May lower total blood cholesterol, LDL ("bad") cholesterol, as well as triglyceride levels.
- May enhance weight-loss efforts.

FORMS

- Capsule
- Tablet
- Softgel
- Liquid

▼ WHAT IT IS

Chromium is a trace mineral that comes in several chemical forms. Supplements usually contain chromium picolinate or chromium polynicotinate. Another type of chromium called chromium dinicotinic acid glutathione is found in brewer's yeast. Supplements may be worthwhile because many people today don't get enough chromium in their diet.

▼ WHAT IT DOES

Chromium helps the body use insulin, a hormone that transfers blood sugar (glucose) to the cells, where it is burned as fuel. With enough chromium, the body can use insulin efficiently and maintain normal blood sugar levels. Chromium also aids the body as it breaks down protein and fat.

PREVENTION
Getting sufficient chromium may prevent diabetes in people with insulin resistance. This disorder makes the body less sensitive to the effects of insulin, so the pancreas has to produce more and more of it to keep blood sugar levels in check. When the pancreas can no longer keep up with the body's demand for extra insulin, type 2 diabetes develops. Chromium may help avert this progression by aiding the body in using insulin more effectively in the first place.

Chromium also helps break down fats, so it may reduce LDL ("bad") and increase HDL ("good") cholesterol levels, lowering the risk of heart disease.

ADDITIONAL BENEFITS
Chromium may relieve headaches, irritability, and other symptoms of low blood sugar (hypoglycemia) by keeping blood sugar levels from dropping below normal. In people with diabetes, it may help control blood sugar levels.

The mineral's most controversial claims relate to weight loss and muscle building. Though some studies indicate that large doses of chromium picolinate can aid in weight reduction or increase muscle mass, others have found no benefit. At best, the mineral may give you a slight edge in weight loss when combined with a sensible diet and regular exercise. But more research is needed to determine chromium's role in this regard.

 ALERT

CAUTION
- People with diabetes should consult their physician before taking chromium. This mineral may alter the dosage of insulin or other diabetes medications.

- **Reminder:** If you have a medical condition, talk to your doctor before taking supplements.

▼ HOW MUCH YOU NEED

No RDA has been established for chromium, but scientists believe that 50 to 200 mcg a day can prevent a deficiency. (Even on a healthy, varied diet, getting the high end of this recommendation would be difficult.)

IF YOU GET TOO LITTLE
A chromium deficiency can lead to inefficient use of glucose. In itself, a lack of chromium is probably not a cause of diabetes, but it can help precipitate the disease in those who are prone to it.

In addition, anxiety, poor metabolism of amino acids, and high blood levels of triglycerides and cholesterol may occur in individuals who don't get enough chromium.

IF YOU GET TOO MUCH
Chromium does not seem to have any adverse effects, although there is some concern that megadoses can impair the absorption of iron and zinc. To compensate for reduced absorption, be sure to get plenty of iron and zinc through your diet or supplements.

▼ HOW TO TAKE IT

DOSAGE
Chromium supplements are generally available in 200 mcg doses.

For general good health: Take 50 to 100 mcg a day, an amount often found in a good multivitamin.
As an aid to a weight-loss program: Take 200 mcg twice a day.
To improve the effectiveness of insulin: Take 200 mcg three times a day.

GUIDELINES FOR USE
• Take chromium in 200 mcg doses with food or a full glass of water to decrease stomach irritation.

• Chromium is better absorbed when combined with foods high in vitamin C (or taken with a vitamin C supplement).

• Both calcium carbonate supplements and antacids can reduce chromium absorption, so don't take them at the same time.

• Don't be confused by labels that suggest that one type of chromium (whether picolinate or polynicotinate) is absorbed better than any other. No reliable research supports these claims.

▼ OTHER SOURCES

Chromium is found in whole grains, whole grain breads and cereals, potatoes, prunes, peanut butter, nuts, seafood, and brewer's yeast. Low-fat diets tend to be higher in chromium than high-fat ones.

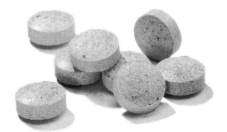
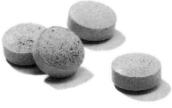

CASE HISTORY

Chromium to the Rescue
A decade after being diagnosed with diabetes, Sarah P. was facing insulin injections because her pills were not effectively regulating her blood sugar. "I felt that if I had to take insulin, I would," she recalls. "But when I read about chromium, I thought, 'Why not try it first?'" Her doctor was concerned and a bit skeptical, but he agreed.

The results didn't occur overnight. "It may seem silly," Sarah says, "but I wanted the chromium to work so much I also began paying extra attention to my diet and forcing myself to take brisk walks twice a day."

Was the chromium what finally reduced her blood sugar to healthier levels? Nobody knows for sure. Sarah's doctor, who read the chromium material Sarah regularly left on his desk, acknowledges he may have dismissed it too soon and would like to see more research done.

Sarah herself is convinced of chromium's benefits. "Sure, I've lost a little weight, but I'm still the same person. My blood sugar hasn't been out of control for months. That's the chromium."

DID YOU KNOW?
Whole grain bread is a good source of chromium. Refined grains, found in white bread, contain little of this essential mineral.

COENZYME Q$_{10}$

Touted as a wonder supplement, coenzyme Q$_{10}$ is reputed to enhance stamina, increase weight loss, combat cancer and AIDS, and even stave off aging. Although these claims may be extravagant, this nutrient does show promise for treating a number of conditions, ranging from heart disease to weak gums.

COMMON USES

■ Improves the symptoms of hypertension and heart disease.

■ Treats gum disease.

■ Protects the nerves and may help slow Alzheimer's or Parkinson's disease.

■ May help prevent cancer, heart disease, and degenerative changes that occur with age.

■ May slow the progression of AIDS or cancer.

FORMS

■ Capsule

■ Softgel

■ Tablet

■ Liquid

▼ WHAT IT IS

Coenzyme Q$_{10}$, a natural substance produced by the body, belongs to a family of compounds called quinones. When it was first isolated in 1957, scientists called it ubiquinone, because it is ubiquitous in nature. In fact, coenzyme Q$_{10}$ is found in all living creatures and is also concentrated in many foods, including nuts and oils.

In the past decade, coenzyme Q$_{10}$ has become one of the most popular dietary supplements around the world. Proponents of the nutrient use it to maintain general good health, as well as to treat heart disease and a number of other serious conditions. Some clinicians believe it is so important for normal body functioning that it should be dubbed "vitamin Q."

▼ WHAT IT DOES

The primary function of coenzyme Q$_{10}$ is as a catalyst for metabolism—the complex chain of chemical reactions during which food is broken down into packets of energy that the body can use. Acting in conjunction with enzymes (hence the name "coenzyme"), the compound speeds up the vital metabolic process, providing the energy that the cells need to digest food, heal wounds, maintain healthy muscles, and perform countless other bodily functions.

Because of the nutrient's essential role in energy production, it's not surprising that it is found in every cell in the body. It is especially abundant in the energy-intensive cells of the heart, helping this organ beat more than 100,000 times each day.

In addition, coenzyme Q$_{10}$ acts as an antioxidant, much like vitamins C and E, helping to neutralize the cell-damaging molecules known as free radicals.

PREVENTION

Coenzyme Q$_{10}$ may play a role in preventing cancer, heart attacks, and other diseases linked to free-radical damage. It's also used as a general energy enhancer and anti-aging

 ALERT

SIDE EFFECTS

• Most research suggests that coenzyme Q$_{10}$ is very safe overall, even in large doses.

• In rare cases, it may cause gastrointestinal symptoms, such as upset stomach, diarrhea, nausea, or loss of appetite.

CAUTION

• Avoid intense exercise while taking coenzyme Q$_{10}$; the heart muscle may become unduly strained or fatigued.

• Pregnant or breast-feeding women should be especially vigilant about checking with their doctor before using coenzyme Q$_{10}$; the nutrient has not been well studied in this group.

• **Reminder:** If you have a medical condition, talk to your doctor before taking supplements.

supplement. Because levels of the compound diminish with age (and with certain diseases), some doctors recommend daily supplementation beginning at about age 40.

MAJOR BENEFITS

Coenzyme Q_{10} has generated much excitement as a possible therapy for heart disease, especially congestive heart failure or a weakened heart. In some studies, patients with a poorly functioning heart have been found to improve greatly after adding the supplement to their conventional drugs and therapies. Other studies have shown that people with cardiovascular disease have low levels of this substance in their heart.

Further research suggests that coenzyme Q_{10} may help protect against blood clots, lower high blood pressure, diminish irregular heartbeats, treat mitral valve prolapse, and relieve chest pains (angina).

If you have heart disease, talk with your doctor about taking this supplement. And remember: Coenzyme Q_{10} is intended as a complement to—and not as a replacement for—conventional medical treatments. Do not take this nutrient in place of heart drugs or other prescribed medications.

ADDITIONAL BENEFITS

A few small studies suggest that coenzyme Q_{10} may prolong survival in those with breast or prostate cancer, though results remain inconclusive. It also appears to aid healing and reduce pain and bleeding in those with gum disease, and to speed recovery following oral surgery.

The supplement shows some promise against Parkinson's and Alzheimer's diseases and fibromyalgia, and it may improve stamina in those with AIDS. Certain practitioners believe the nutrient helps stabilize blood sugar levels in people with diabetes.

There are many other claims made for the supplement: that it slows aging, aids weight loss, enhances athletic performance, combats chronic fatigue syndrome, relieves multiple allergies, and boosts immunity. But more research is needed to determine the effectiveness of coenzyme Q_{10} for these and other conditions.

▼ HOW TO TAKE IT

DOSAGE

The general dosage is 50 mg twice a day. Higher dosages of 100 mg twice a day may be useful for heart or circulatory disorders, or for Alzheimer's disease and other specific complaints.

GUIDELINES FOR USE

• Take a supplement morning and evening, preferably with food to enhance absorption.

• Coenzyme Q_{10} should be continued long term; it may require eight weeks or longer to notice results.

SHOPPING HINTS

■ Although coenzyme Q_{10} is widespread in nature, it is not cheap to buy. A typical daily dose of 100 mg can cost about $40 a month. Shop around a bit or try a mail-order vitamin supplier to get the lowest price.

■ Look for capsules or tablets that contain coenzyme Q_{10} in an oil base (soybean or another oil). Because it is a fat-soluble compound, this nutrient is best absorbed when taken with food.

LATEST FINDINGS

■ In a major study in Italy of more than 2,500 patients with congestive heart failure, 80% showed improvement when a daily dose of 100 mg of coenzyme Q_{10} was added to their other treatment. They had better color and less ankle swelling (edema) and shortness of breath. They also slept better after taking the supplement for 90 days.

DID YOU KNOW?

Doctors commonly prescribe coenzyme Q_{10} to treat heart disease in Japan, Sweden, Italy, Canada, and other countries. Many of the supplement preparations are made in Japan, a country where up to 1 in 10 adults takes coenzyme Q_{10} regularly.

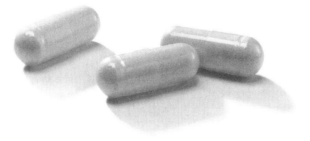

COPPER

Essential in preventing cardiovascular disease, maintaining healthy skin and hair color, and promoting fertility, copper is the least discussed but third most abundant trace mineral in the human body. Even so, some experts now believe that many people may be marginally deficient in this important nutrient.

COMMON USES

■ Strengthens blood vessels, bones, tendons, and nerves.

■ Helps maintain fertility.

■ Ensures healthy pigmentation of hair and skin.

■ Promotes blood clotting.

FORMS

■ Tablet

■ Capsule

▼ WHAT IT IS

Copper, the reddish brown malleable metal commonly used in cookware and plumbing, is also found in at least 15 proteins in the human body. This mineral is available in nutritional supplement form as copper aspartate, copper citrate, and copper picolinate.

Although it can be obtained from a wide variety of foods, the typical American diet is low in copper, because the foods that are the best sources, such as oysters and liver, are not eaten frequently.

▼ WHAT IT DOES

Copper is essential in the formation of collagen, a fundamental protein in bones, skin, and connective tissue. It also may help the body use its stored iron and play a role in maintaining immunity and fertility.

Involved in the formation of melanin (a dark natural color found in the hair, skin, and eyes), copper promotes consistent pigmentation as well.

PREVENTION

Evidence suggests that copper can be a factor in preventing high blood pressure and heart rhythm disorders (arrhythmias). And some experts believe that it may protect tissues from damage by free radicals, helping to prevent cancer, heart disease, and other ailments. Getting enough copper may also help keep cholesterol levels low.

ADDITIONAL BENEFITS

Copper is necessary for the manufacture of many enzymes, especially superoxide dismutase (SOD), which appears to be one of the body's most potent antioxidants. It may also help stave off the bone loss that can lead to osteoporosis.

▼ HOW MUCH YOU NEED

Although there is no daily RDA for copper, adults are advised to obtain 1.5 to 3 mg daily to keep the body functioning normally.

IF YOU GET TOO LITTLE

A true copper deficiency is rare. It usually occurs only in individuals with illnesses such as Crohn's disease or celiac disease or in those with inherited conditions that inhibit copper absorption, such as albinism. Symptoms of deficiency are fatigue; heart

 ALERT

CAUTION

• It's important to take extra copper when using zinc for longer than a month, because zinc interferes with the body's ability to absorb copper.

• **Reminder:** If you have a medical condition, talk to your doctor before taking supplements.

rhythm disorders; brittle, discolored hair; high blood pressure; skeletal defects; and infertility.

But even a mild deficiency may have some adverse health effects. For example, a preliminary study involving 24 men found that a diet low in copper caused a significant increase in LDL ("bad") cholesterol as well as a decrease in HDL ("good") cholesterol. These changes in their cholesterol profiles increased the participants' risk of heart disease.

IF YOU GET TOO MUCH

Just 10 mg of copper taken at one time can produce nausea, muscle pain, and stomachache. Severe copper toxicity from oral copper supplements has not been noted to date. However, some people who work with pesticides containing copper have suffered liver damage, coma, and even death.

▼ HOW TO TAKE IT

DOSAGE

Though there is no need to consume megadoses of copper, it is preferable to get amounts in the upper range of the recommended intake (3 mg a day from food and supplements combined).

Most good multivitamins will contain 1 mg copper, meeting nearly half the daily requirement.

GUIDELINES FOR USE

• It is advisable to take a supplement at the same time every day, preferably with a meal to decrease the chance of stomach irritation.

• If you take zinc supplements for longer than one month, add 2 mg of copper to your regimen. People who take antacids regularly may need extra copper as well.

▼ OTHER SOURCES

Shellfish (oysters, lobsters, crabs) and organ meats (liver) are excellent sources of copper. However, if you're concerned about your cholesterol levels, there are many vegetarian foods rich in copper as well. These include legumes; whole grains, such as rye and wheat, and products made from them (bread, cereal, pasta); nuts and seeds; vegetables such as peas, artichokes, avocados, radishes, garlic, mushrooms, and potatoes; fruits such as tomatoes, bananas, and prunes; and soy products (tofu, tempeh, soy milk, and soy powder).

SHOPPING HINTS

■ Individual copper supplements may be hard to find at the pharmacy or health-food store. This mineral is more commonly sold in combination with zinc.

■ Ignore the label claims that one particular form of copper is better for you than another. There is no evidence that any one form (copper aspartate, copper citrate, or copper picolinate) is better absorbed than another or otherwise preferred by the body.

LATEST FINDINGS

■ Copper may help prevent osteoporosis. In a recent study involving healthy women ages 45 to 56, those taking a daily 3 mg copper supplement showed no loss in mineral bone density, but women given a placebo showed a significant loss.

DID YOU KNOW?

You'd have to eat about 6 medium avocados to get the 3 mg of copper you need each day.

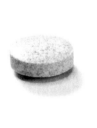
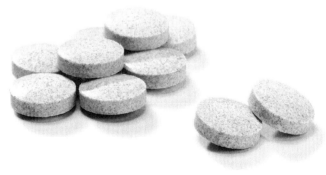

CRANBERRY *(Vaccinium macrocarpon)*

These tangy, ruby red berries, native to the New World and now such an integral part of the American Thanksgiving tradition, have long been considered nature's cure for the urinary tract infections that frequently plague women of all ages. Modern science has now confirmed that this folk wisdom has real merit.

COMMON USES

■ Treats lower urinary tract infections (commonly referred to as bladder infections or cystitis).

■ May prevent recurrence of urinary tract infections.

■ Helps deodorize urine.

FORMS

■ Capsule

■ Tablet

■ Softgel

■ Liquid/Juice

■ Fresh or dried fruit

■ Tea

▼ WHAT IT IS

The cranberry, an indigenous American plant closely related to the blueberry, has been used for centuries in both healing and cooking. The name is a shortened form of craneberry—the flowers of the low-growing shrub were thought to resemble the heads of the cranes that frequented the bogs where it grew. The berries are now widely cultivated throughout the United States, especially in Massachusetts and Washington state.

In early American medicine, cranberries were crushed and used as poultices for treating wounds and tumors, and also as a remedy for scurvy, a gum and bleeding disorder caused by a deficiency of vitamin C. In this century, medicinal interest in cranberry has focused on its important role in preventing and treating urinary tract infections (UTIs), which are caused by *E. coli* and other types of bacteria.

▼ WHAT IT DOES

In the 1920s, it was discovered that people who consumed large amounts of cranberries produced a more acidic urine, and that the urine was purified in the process. During this purification process, a powerful substance called hippuric acid was created. It proved to have a strong antibiotic effect on the urinary tract. In fact, it discouraged and sometimes even eliminated the harmful infection-causing bacteria.

More recent studies, however, indicate that cranberry's main infection-fighting capabilities may be due to a different property: Cranberry appears to inhibit the adhesion of harmful microorganisms to certain cells lining the urinary tract. This makes the environment a less hospitable place for *E. coli* and other bacteria to replicate, and thus reduces the likelihood of infection.

Scientists have isolated two substances that produce this effect. One is fructose, a sugar that is found in many fruit juices. The other is a poorly understood compound present in cranberry

 ALERT

SIDE EFFECTS

• There are no known side effects from either the short-term or long-term use of cranberry. Cranberry appears to be safe for pregnant and breastfeeding women.

CAUTION

• Cranberry is not a substitute for antibiotics during an acute urinary tract infection (UTI). See your doctor if you don't feel better after 24 to 36 hours of using cranberry for a suspected UTI.

• See your doctor right away if symptoms include fever, chills, back pain, or blood in the urine, which may be signs of a kidney infection (upper UTI) requiring medical attention.

• If you are at risk for kidney stones, opt for cranberry juice rather than tablet or capsules, which can be highly concentrated.

• **Reminder:** If you have a medical condition, talk to your doctor before taking supplements.

and blueberry juices but absent from grapefruit, orange, guava, mango, and pineapple juices.

MAJOR BENEFITS

Scientists have now confirmed the effectiveness of cranberry in preventing and treating UTIs. Several studies have shown that daily consumption of cranberry, either in juice or capsule form, dramatically reduces the recurrence of UTIs. Women are 10 times more likely to develop these infections than men—in fact, 25% to 35% of women ages 20 to 40 have had at least one. There's no reason, however, why men can't benefit from taking cranberry as well.

Cranberry also appears to shorten the course of urinary tract illness, helping to alleviate pain, burning, itching, and other symptoms. It's important to remember, though, that persistent UTIs should be treated promptly with antibiotics to prevent more serious complications. However, cranberry juice can be safely taken along with conventional drugs. It may even help hasten healing.

ADDITIONAL BENEFITS

Because it helps deodorize urine, cranberry should be in the diet of anyone suffering from the embarrassing odors associated with incontinence. In addition, cranberry's high vitamin C content makes it a natural vitamin supplement.

▼ HOW TO TAKE IT

DOSAGE

To help treat urinary tract infections: You should get about 800 mg of cranberry extract a day (two 400 mg pills). Or you can drink at least 16 ounces of undiluted juice a day or take it in liquid extract form (follow the package directions).
To prevent recurrences: The dose for an infection can be cut in half, to 400 mg of cranberry a day.

GUIDELINES FOR USE

• Cranberry can be taken with or without food. Drinking plenty of water or other fluids along with cranberry and throughout the day should also help to speed recovery.

• Cranberry has no known interactions with antibiotics or other medications. But by acidifying the urine, cranberry may lessen the effect of another herb called uva ursi (also known as bearberry) that is sometimes used for UTIs. Try one or the other herb, but don't take them in combination.

SHOPPING HINTS

■ For best medical effect, choose cranberry capsules or undiluted juice (which contains higher concentrations of the active ingredients) over presweetened juice. The processed commercial product (cranberry juice cocktail) is only one-third cranberry juice.

■ High-quality undiluted cranberry juice is sold at health-food stores. To make it more palatable, add sugar or other sweeteners to taste.

LATEST FINDINGS

■ A major study in the *Journal of the American Medical Association* looked at 153 elderly women (average age 78) who had no urinary tract symptoms. Half the women drank 300 ml (about a cup) of undiluted cranberry juice every day, and the other half received a placebo. After four to eight weeks, those who drank the cranberry juice were much less prone to urinary tract infections and had lower levels of potentially harmful bacteria in their urine.

■ Research confirms that cranberry is effective for younger as well as older women. In a study in Utah, women ages 28 to 44 who took cranberry capsules (400 mg a day) for three months were only 40% as likely to have a UTI as women who were given a placebo.

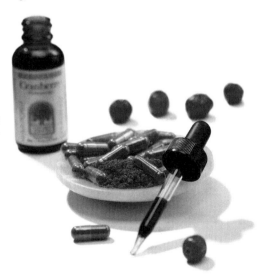

The common cranberry is a source of extracts in liquid and capsule form; both are effective for urinary tract infections.

DANDELION *(Taraxacum officinale)*

Known mostly as a prolific wild weed whose yellow flower dots lawns and roadsides all over the United States, dandelion is grown commercially in Europe. This is because its leaves and roots are a rich source of vitamins and minerals, and its active ingredients are particularly useful for treating digestive and liver problems.

COMMON USES

■ Bolsters the liver; useful during cases of hepatitis (liver inflammation) and jaundice.

■ Aids digestion by stimulating release of bile from the liver and gallbladder; may help prevent gallstones.

■ Helps treat endometriosis.

■ Boosts iron absorption to combat some cases of anemia.

FORMS

■ Capsule

■ Tablet

■ Liquid/Juice

■ Dried or fresh herb/Tea

▼ WHAT IT IS

Dandelion grows wild throughout much of the world and is cultivated in parts of Europe for medicinal uses. Closely related to chicory, this perennial plant can grow up to a foot high; its spatula-shaped leaves are shiny, hairless, and deeply toothed.

The solitary yellow flower blooms for much of the growing season, opening at daybreak and closing at dusk and in wet weather (some cultures have used dandelions to signal the approach of rain). After the flower matures, the plant forms a puffball of seeds that are dispersed by the wind (or by the antics of playful children).

Supplements usually contain the herb's root (which is tapered and sweet to the taste) or leaves, though the whole plant and its flowers are also valued for their healing properties.

▼ WHAT IT DOES

Folk healers have long prescribed dandelion for liver and digestive problems. Because its various active ingredients enhance the performance of the liver, this herb is useful for treating a wide range of disorders.

MAJOR BENEFITS

Studies of dandelion's beneficial effects on the liver have shown that the herb increases the production and flow of bile (a digestive aid) from the liver and gallbladder, helping to treat such conditions as gallstones, jaundice, and hepatitis. It is thought that the plant's positive effect on various liver functions is probably related to its high content of the B vitamin choline.

Dandelion is sometimes mixed with other nutritional supplements that bolster liver function, including milk thistle, black radish, celandine, beet leaf, fringe tree bark, inositol, methionine, choline, and others. Such combinations are usually sold as liver or lipotropic ("fat-metabolizing") formulas in health-food stores.

Because it improves liver function, dandelion (in combination with other liver-strengthening nutrients) may be effective for relieving the pain and

---

 ALERT

SIDE EFFECTS

• Dandelion has no serious side effects. In large doses, it may cause a skin rash, upset stomach, or diarrhea. Stop using it if this happens, and discuss the reaction with your doctor.

CAUTION

• Dandelion should not be used during acute attacks of gallstones or by people with bile duct problems or a bowel obstruction (often signaled by persistent constipation or lack of bowel movements). Seek professional medical attention.

• **Reminder:** If you have a medical condition, talk to your doctor before taking supplements.

other symptoms of endometriosis. It enhances the ability of the liver to remove excess estrogen from the body, thereby helping to restore a healthy balance of hormones in women who are afflicted with this disorder.

ADDITIONAL BENEFITS

Dandelion root acts as a mild laxative, so a tea made from it may provide a gentle remedy for constipation. The herb may also enhance the body's ability to absorb iron from either food or supplements, which may help combat some cases of anemia.

Some studies also indicate that dandelion may be of value in treating cancer. The Japanese have patented a freeze-dried extract of dandelion root to use against tumors; the Chinese are employing dandelion extracts in fighting breast cancer (a treatment supported by positive effects in animal studies). But additional studies need to be conducted in humans to determine the herb's true effectiveness against specific types of cancer.

As for other medical applications, studies have found that dandelion can lower blood sugar levels in animals, suggesting it may have some role to play in the treatment of diabetes. It may also have some diuretic effects, so it is sometimes given for water retention and bloating.

▼ HOW TO TAKE IT

DOSAGE

To strengthen liver function in hepatitis, gallstones, and endometriosis: Take 500 mg of a powdered solid dandelion root extract twice a day. This amount may also be found in some lipotropic (liver) combinations. Or take 1 teaspoon of a liquid dandelion extract in water three times a day.
For constipation: Drink one cup of dandelion root tea three times a day.
For anemia: Have 1 teaspoon of fresh dandelion juice or tincture each morning and evening with half a glass of water.

GUIDELINES FOR USE

• Drink fresh dandelion juice or liquid extract with water.

• Take pills containing dandelion root extract with or without food.

• Although no adverse effects have been reported in pregnant or breast-feeding women, dandelion preparations may have diuretic effects, so this group of women may want to avoid the herb.

• Don't use dandelions growing in a lawn or yard medicinally. Instead, get them from health-food stores and make sure that they were grown in organic, fertilizer-free soil.

FACTS & TIPS

■ To make dandelion tea, use the dried chopped root or leaves of the dandelion. Pour a cup of very hot (but not boiling) water over 1 or 2 teaspoons of the herb and allow it to steep for about 15 minutes. The tea can be blended with other herbs, such as licorice, and sweetened with honey.

■ Dandelion is a healthful and nutritious food or beverage. Organically grown dandelion leaves and flowers are quite tasty when steamed like spinach, and its pleasantly bitter greens make a tangy addition to salads. A juice can be extracted from the leaves, and the root can be roasted and used to brew a beverage that substitutes for coffee (without the stimulant effects).

DID YOU KNOW?

Dandelion was introduced to the New World by the first English settlers, who grew it in window boxes and herb gardens. Hudson's Bay Company, founded in 1670, exported dandelion roots to its Canadian outposts to supplement the high-meat diet of its overseas employees.

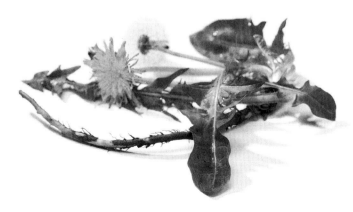

DHEA

Some advocates of the nutritional supplement DHEA call it the fountain of youth. Although the claim may be overblown, this hormone has shown some promise in combating certain age-related diseases. More study is needed, however, to identify the exact effects of DHEA—as well as the people who could benefit most from it.

COMMON USES

- May lower risk of heart disease.
- Aids in glucose management in some people with diabetes.
- Boosts the immune system.
- Relieves some lupus symptoms.
- May help people with HIV/AIDS.

FORMS

- Tablet
- Capsule
- Cream

▼ WHAT IT IS

Nicknamed the "mother of hormones," DHEA, which is scientifically known as dehydroepiandrosterone, is needed by the body to produce many types of hormones, including estrogen and testosterone. DHEA is secreted by the body's two adrenal glands—small organs located on top of the kidneys—as well as by the skin, brain, testicles, and ovaries.

Although women make less DHEA than men, in both sexes DHEA production declines dramatically with age; levels are 80% lower at age 70 than at age 30. The significance of these falling DHEA levels, however, has not been determined.

▼ WHAT IT DOES

There has been plenty of hype surrounding DHEA, so it is difficult to separate wishful thinking from sound scientific evidence. DHEA has been said to stimulate weight loss, increase libido, enhance memory, and prevent osteoporosis. All these claims, however, are unsupported.

Studies do indicate that DHEA may improve general well-being in older people (although just how isn't clear), reduce the risk of heart disease, ease symptoms of the autoimmune disease lupus, help manage diabetes, and bolster immunity.

MAJOR BENEFITS

Having blood levels of DHEA on the high end of normal may lower the risk of heart disease for older men. In one study, men with naturally high DHEA levels had less body fat and higher HDL ("good") cholesterol levels than men with low DHEA levels.

Those with high DHEA levels also did better on an exercise stress test, a procedure that measures the condition of the heart during physical exertion. These associations weren't seen in women, however. In fact, women who took DHEA seemed to have a slightly higher risk of heart disease.

Other research suggests that DHEA may help "thin" the blood and so

  ALERT

SIDE EFFECTS

• When used to excess, DHEA supplements can cause acne, extremely oily skin, hair growth in women, breast enlargement in men, deepening of the voice, and mood changes.

• One animal study demonstrated an association between liver cancer and excessively high doses of DHEA.

CAUTION

• DHEA is a hormone; as such it may be linked to the development of some cancers, such as breast or prostate. Anyone who has these cancers, or is at risk for them, should not use DHEA.

• **Reminder:** If you have a medical condition, talk to your doctor before taking supplements.

reduce the likelihood of blood clot formation and possible heart attack.

Some evidence of DHEA's immune-boosting action was noted in a study of older people who had received flu shots. Their immune response to the weakened flu virus in the injection was significantly increased after taking DHEA. Researchers are now hopeful that DHEA might improve immune responses in people infected with HIV, the virus that causes AIDS.

ADDITIONAL BENEFITS

A small study of postmenopausal women indicated that those taking DHEA had lower levels of triglycerides (a blood fat related to cholesterol) and were able to use insulin more efficiently than women not given DHEA. This finding suggests a possible role for the supplement in the treatment of diabetes.

DHEA has also been reported to have beneficial effects on patients with lupus, an autoimmune disease. It relieved some symptoms and reduced the amount of medication needed.

▼ HOW TO TAKE IT

DOSAGE

DHEA supplements should be taken only to raise hormone levels to within a normal range—not to exceed those levels. Start with a low dose (5 to 10 mg a day for women; 25 mg a day for men) and slowly increase the amount to achieve the desired effect. The maximum dose should not exceed 50 mg a day unless you're using it for a specific disorder, such as lupus or HIV. It's best to take DHEA in the morning. People under age 50 who are healthy don't need the supplement at all.

GUIDELINES FOR USE

• Although DHEA is readily available in health-food stores and vitamin shops, it is more potent than many other nutrients or herbs. And the long-term effects of DHEA supplementation are simply not known. For this reason most experts believe you should take DHEA only under the supervision of a doctor. Therefore try to find a physician who is familiar with the use of this nutritional supplement.

• Before taking DHEA, make sure your doctor checks for prostate cancer (men) or breast cancer (women), because such cancers are influenced by hormone levels in the body.

• Be sure to have a blood test to determine your current DHEA levels and use this supplement only if your blood level of this hormone is low. After three weeks, have another blood test to assess whether your dosage needs adjustment. Once obtained, a satisfactory blood level can often be maintained with as little as 5 to 10 mg of DHEA a week.

SHOPPING HINTS

■ The labels on wild yam products sometimes claim that the herb contains substances that are converted to DHEA or other hormones once within the body. In fact, this conversion can be achieved only in a laboratory, not by the human body.

LATEST FINDINGS

■ Although there's no evidence that DHEA will lengthen your life, it may enhance your quality of life. In a recent study, older men and women taking DHEA reported increased feelings of well-being, improved sleep, more energy, and a greater ability to handle stress. More than 80% of the women and 67% of the men had a positive response to DHEA, compared with less than 10% of the people taking a placebo.

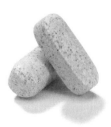

DONG QUAI *(Angelica sinensis, A. acutiloba)*

An ingredient in many herbal "women's supplements," dong quai (also known as angelica) is a traditional tonic used in Asia to aid the female reproductive system. Its popularity is second only to that of ginseng in China and Japan, but Western experts continue to debate the effectiveness of this ancient herb.

COMMON USES

- May help ease menstrual cramps.
- May reduce hot flashes associated with menopause.

FORMS

- Capsule
- Tablet
- Softgel
- Tincture
- Liquid
- Dried herb/Tea

▼ WHAT IT IS

Although dong quai grows wild in Asia, it's also widely cultivated for medicinal purposes in China (the *Angelica sinensis* variety) and in Japan (*A. acutiloba*), where many women take it daily to maintain overall good health.

The most widely available therapeutic form is derived from the root of *A. sinensis*, a plant with hollow stems that grows up to eight feet tall and has clusters of white flowers. When it's in bloom, angelica resembles Queen Anne's lace, its botanical relative.

Other common names for dong quai include dang gui, tang kuie, and Chinese angelica.

▼ WHAT IT DOES

Generally, dong quai is believed to keep the uterus healthy and to regulate the menstrual cycle. It may also widen blood vessels and increase blood flow to various organs. Even among herbal experts, however, questions linger about its benefits. One reason it has been difficult to assess is that it's often taken along with other herbs.

MAJOR BENEFITS

Traditionally, dong quai has been used for menstrual and menopausal difficulties. Claims for the herb include balancing the menstrual cycle, correcting abnormal bleeding patterns, alleviating symptoms of premenstrual syndrome (PMS), easing menstrual cramps, reducing menopausal hot flashes, and improving the vaginal dryness sometimes associated with menopause.

There are two theories about how dong quai may help relieve these problems. Some herbalists believe it contains plant estrogens (phytoestrogens); these are weaker than estrogens produced by the body but they do chemically bind with estrogen receptors in human cells. Because of this, phytoestrogens may minimize the potential negative effects of a woman's own estrogen, which can include an increased risk of breast cancer.

Phytoestrogens also may prevent hot flashes by compensating for the

 ALERT

SIDE EFFECTS

- Dong quai may have a mild laxative effect and may promote heavy menstrual bleeding.

- Dong quai may increase your skin's sensitivity to the sun, resulting in rashes or severe sunburns.

CAUTION

- Dong quai should not be used by pregnant women or mothers who are breast-feeding.

- People on anticoagulants (blood-thinners) or NSAIDs (nonsteroidal anti-inflammatory drugs) should not take dong quai without consulting a doctor.

- **Reminder:** If you have a medical condition, talk to your doctor before taking supplements.

decline in estrogen levels that occurs after menopause.

Other experts attribute the effectiveness of dong quai to its abundance of coumarins. This group of natural chemicals dilates blood vessels, increases blood flow to the uterus and other organs, and stimulates the central nervous system. Coumarins also appear to reduce inflammation and muscle spasms, which may account for dong quai's ability to reduce the severity of menstrual cramps.

ADDITIONAL BENEFITS
Although dong quai is not typically used to lower blood pressure, it does have this effect because it dilates blood vessels, making it easier for the heart to pump blood through the body. The herb is also rich in vitamin B_{12}, and so may help build red blood cells.

▼ HOW TO TAKE IT

DOSAGE
For PMS, menstrual irregularities, menstrual cramps, or hot flashes: Take 600 mg of dong quai daily. This is also available from 30 drops (1.5 ml) of tincture three times

a day. In either pill or liquid form, extracts should be standardized to contain 0.8% to 1.1% ligustilide. You can also use a single preparation in which dong quai is combined with menstrual-regulating herbs. Such herbs include chasteberry, licorice, and Siberian ginseng.

GUIDELINES FOR USE
• *For symptoms of PMS,* use dong quai only on the days that you are not menstruating.
• *For menstrual cramps with PMS,* continue using dong quai until menstruation stops.
• *For cramps without PMS,* begin taking dong quai the day before your period is due.
• *For hot flashes,* use dong quai daily. Continue the herb for two months before deciding if it works.

• Protect yourself from the sun when using dong quai, because the plant's root contains compounds called psoralens that can make some people more sensitive to sunlight and cause a rash or severe sunburn.

SHOPPING HINTS

■ If you want to try dong quai for menstrual cramps or menopausal symptoms, make sure to purchase Chinese or Japanese angelica (*Angelica sinensis* or *A. acutiloba*). Traditionally, the American and European angelicas (*A. archangelica* or *A. atropurpurea*) have both been widely used for respiratory ailments and stomach upset, but these species have shown no real effect for gynecological problems.

LATEST FINDINGS

■ A recent study found dong quai was no better than a placebo as a remedy for hot flashes and other menopausal problems, such as vaginal dryness. Both dong quai and the placebo reduced the frequency of hot flashes by 25% to 30%. But this study tested the effect of dong quai alone. In Asia, it is traditionally used in combination with other herbs.

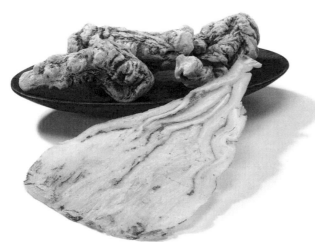

Dong quai's naturally gnarled root is flattened out for medicinal use.

ECHINACEA *(Echinacea angustifolia, E. purpurea, E. pallida)*

Long used by Native Americans, midwestern settlers, and earlier generations of doctors, this herb which grows wild on the American prairies fell out of favor with the advent of modern antibiotics. But echinacea is regaining popularity as a safe and powerful immune-system booster to fight colds, flu, and other infections.

COMMON USES
- Reduces susceptibility to colds/flu.
- Limits duration/severity of infections.
- Helps fight recurrent respiratory, middle ear, urinary tract, and vaginal yeast infections.
- Speeds the healing of skin wounds and inflammations.

FORMS
- Capsule
- Tablet
- Softgel
- Lozenge
- Tincture/Liquid
- Dried herb/Tea

▼ WHAT IT IS

Also known as the purple, or prairie, coneflower, echinacea (pronounced ek-in-NAY-sha) is a wildflower with daisylike purple blossoms that is native to the grasslands of the central United States. For centuries, the Plains tribes used the plant to heal wounds and to counteract the toxins of snakebites. The herb also became popular with European-American pioneers and their physicians, who considered it an all-purpose infection fighter.

Of the nine echinacea species, three (*Echinacea angustifolia, E. pallida,* and *E. purpurea*) are used medicinally. They appear in literally hundreds of commercial preparations, which utilize different parts of the plant (flowers, leaves, stems, or roots) and come in a variety of forms. Echinacea contains many active ingredients that are thought to strengthen the immune system, and in recent years, it has become one of the most popular herbal remedies in the world.

▼ WHAT IT DOES

A natural antibiotic and infection fighter, echinacea helps to kill bacteria, viruses, fungi, and other disease-causing microbes. It acts by stimulating various immune-system cells that are key weapons against infection. In addition, the herb boosts the cells' production of an innate virus-fighting substance called interferon. Because these effects are relatively shortlived, however, the herb is best administered at frequent intervals—as often as every couple of hours during acute infections.

PREVENTION
Echinacea can help prevent the two most common viral ailments—colds and flu. It is most effective when taken at the first hint of illness. In one study of people who were susceptible to colds, those who used the herb for eight weeks were 35% less likely to come down with a cold than those given a placebo. Furthermore, they caught colds less often—40 days elapsed between infections, versus 25 days for the placebo group.

ALERT

SIDE EFFECTS
- At recommended doses, echinacea has no known side effects.
- People who are allergic to daisylike flowers may also be allergic to echinacea. If you develop a skin rash or breathing problems, call your doctor.

CAUTION
- If you're taking antibiotics or other drugs for an infection, use echinacea as an addition to, not as a replacement for, those medications.
- Echinacea can overstimulate the immune system and may worsen symptoms of lupus, multiple sclerosis, rheumatoid arthritis, or other autoimmune disorders. It may also be counterproductive in progressive infections such as tuberculosis.
- Because the risks remain unclear, women who are trying to conceive, or who are pregnant or breast-feeding, should avoid using echinacea.
- **Reminder:** If you have a medical condition, talk to your doctor before taking supplements.

Studies confirm that echinacea is also useful if you're already suffering from the aches, pains, congestion, or fever of colds or flu. Overall, symptoms are less severe and subside sooner.

ADDITIONAL BENEFITS

Echinacea may be of value for recurrent ailments, including vaginal yeast, urinary tract, and middle ear infections. It is also sometimes used to treat strep throat, staph infections, herpes infections (including genital herpes, cold sores, and shingles), bronchitis, and sinus infections. Moreover, the herb is being studied as a possible treatment for chronic fatigue syndrome and AIDS. And it may prove effective against some types of cancer, particularly in patients whose immune systems are depressed by radiation or chemotherapy.

Echinacea can be applied to the skin as well. Its juice promotes the healing of all kinds of wounds, boils, eczema, abscesses, burns, canker or cold sores, and bedsores. To treat a sore throat or tonsillitis, the tincture can be diluted and used as a gargle.

▼ HOW TO TAKE IT

DOSAGE

Because echinacea comes in many different forms, check the product's label for the proper dosage.

For colds and flu: A high dose is needed—up to 200 mg five a times a day. In one major study, patients with the flu who were given 900 mg of echinacea a day did better than those who received either a lower dosage of 450 mg a day or a placebo.

For other infections: The recommended dose is 200 mg three or four times a day.

For long-term use as a general immune booster: To derive the most benefits, especially for those prone to chronic infections, alternate echinacea every three weeks with other immune-enhancing herbs, including goldenseal, astragalus, pau d'arco, and medicinal mushrooms. Echinacea teas, often blended with other herbs, are available as well.

GUIDELINES FOR USE

• Echinacea should be used no longer than eight weeks, followed by a one-week interval before you resume taking it. Some studies suggest that with continuous use, the herb's immunity-boosting effects diminish. Starting and stopping, or rotating it with other herbs, may maximize its effectiveness. You can take echinacea with or without food.

• Check the alcohol content of echinacea tinctures; many contain considerable amounts of alcohol, making them unsuitable for children and for people with liver disease or alcoholism.

SHOPPING HINTS

■ Buying echinacea can be confusing because it comes in many different forms. Experts often recommend a liquid—the fresh-pressed juice (standardized to contain 2.4% beta-1, 2-fructofuranosides), a liquid extract, or an alcohol-based tincture (containing a 5:1 concentration). Those who dislike the bitter taste of the liquids can take standardized extracts in pill form. Look for pills containing at least 3.5% echinacosides.

LATEST FINDINGS

■ In a recent study in Germany, a small group of patients with advanced colon cancer received echinacea along with standard chemotherapy. The herb appeared to prolong survival in these patients, presumably by boosting the immune system's ability to fight cancer cells. Additional research is needed to define the possible role of this herb in combating colon and other forms of cancer.

DID YOU KNOW?

Echinacea contains a substance that makes the lips and tongue tingle when taken in liquid form. If you use a liquid preparation, look for this effect—it's often a good indication that you've bought a high-quality product.

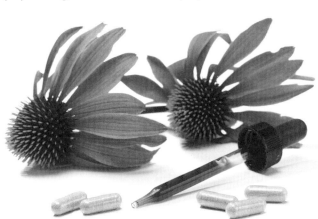

EPHEDRA *(Ephedra sinica, E. intermedia, E. equisetina)*

Sometimes called the world's oldest medicine, this herb has been used in China to treat colds and asthma since ancient times, probably as early as 3000 B.C. It's still considered an effective remedy for bronchial disorders, but concerns about its abuse and safety have made ephedra controversial in recent years.

COMMON USES

■ Eases congestion and labored breathing due to allergies or asthma.

■ Relieves pressure and congestion in sinus infections (sinusitis).

■ May aid weight loss.

FORMS

■ Capsule

■ Tablet

■ Liquid

■ Dried herb/Tea

 ## WHAT IT IS

Also known by its Chinese name *Ma huang,* ephedra is made from the dried stems of *Ephedra sinica,* a shrub native to desert regions of Asia. However, preparations from species such as *E. intermedia* or *E. equisetina* may also be effective. A synthetic version of ephedra's active ingredients is widely used in both prescription and over-the-counter drugs, including hundreds of cold, allergy, asthma, weight-loss, and energy-boosting formulas.

Unfortunately, the herb has been abused in recent years, when some people began taking very high doses as a recreational stimulant—leading to heart attacks, strokes, and numerous deaths. As a result, the FDA has considered banning the supplement. Though a ban has not been imposed, the FDA has proposed that all ephedra preparations carry a warning label.

WHAT IT DOES

Ephedra's primary active ingredients, the chemicals ephedrine and pseudoephedrine, have two major effects: They stimulate the central nervous system and they open the airways.

Ephedra's stimulant effect is stronger than that of caffeine, but less potent than that of amphetamines or of the natural adrenal hormone epinephrine (adrenaline), which prepares the body for stressful situations (the "fight-or-flight" response). Ephedra makes the heart beat faster, increases blood pressure, speeds up the metabolism, and acts as a diuretic.

But throughout ephedra's long history, its main use has been as a bronchodilator, used to treat the bronchial and nasal congestion of asthma, allergies, colds, and sinus infections. In the 1920s, U.S. drug companies began extracting active ingredients from the herb and using it in asthma and cold

 ## ALERT

SIDE EFFECTS

• The higher the dose and the longer you take ephedra, the greater the risk for such common side effects as nervousness, insomnia, heart palpitations, and paleness.

• Less common side effects of ephedra include dizziness, tingling, nausea and vomiting, loss of appetite, muscle cramps, headache, and difficult or painful urination.

• Extremely serious reactions include high blood pressure, stroke, seizures, and with very high doses, hallucinations and psychosis.

CAUTION

• Don't exceed recommended daily dosages. And be sure to factor in amounts from other sources, such as over-the-counter cold remedies.

• Ephedra can cause blood pressure to soar. Check with your doctor before taking ephedra if you have high blood pressure, heart disease, or a heart rhythm disorder, or take an MAO inhibitor drug. Also at risk for complications are people with kidney disease or a history of seizures.

• Talk to your doctor if you have diabetes, thyroid disease, difficulty urinating due to prostate problems, or are pregnant or breast-feeding.

• **Reminder:** If you have a medical problem, talk to your doctor before taking supplements.

medicines—a practice that many companies still follow today.

MAJOR BENEFITS

Ephedra dilates the small airways in the lungs (the bronchioles), thus relieving congestion and coughing due to seasonal allergies or to mild asthma. Ephedra also plays a role in alleviating respiratory symptoms caused by colds, flu, and sinus infections.

ADDITIONAL BENEFITS

Some weight-loss supplements claim that ephedra, usually in combination with St. John's wort, is an "herbal fen-phen," a natural alternative to the antiobesity prescription drugs fenfluramine (now banned for possibly causing heart disease) and phentermine. Though ephedra may make the body burn calories quickly and suppress appetite, studies of this herb as a weight-loss aid have been contradictory. For those in otherwise good health, it may be safe and effective in recommended doses.

More controversial is the claim that ephedra enhances athletic performance by boosting energy. Not only is there no scientific basis for this theory, but it has had tragic consequences: A number of athletes have become seriously ill—and several have died—after taking large doses of products containing ephedra. The herb is currently listed as a banned substance by the U.S. Olympic Committee.

▼ HOW TO TAKE IT

DOSAGE

Check your bottle's label to see how much ephedrine is contained in each dose of ephedra. Most standardized extracts supply about 5.5% to 6.5%

ephedrine (also known as "ephedra alkaloids"). Begin with a low daily dose, such as 100 mg of ephedra (about 6 mg of ephedrine). If side effects aren't a problem, increase the dose, but don't exceed 130 mg of ephedra (about 8 mg of ephedrine) three times a day. Don't take more than 8 mg ephedra every six hours.

To make a tea, pour one cup of very hot water over 1 teaspoon of dried ephedra (along with other herbs if desired); steep for 10 to 15 minutes. Drink one or two cups a day. Or take ¼ to 1 teaspoon ephedra liquid extract (up to 8 mg of ephedrine) in a glass of water up to three times daily.

GUIDELINES FOR USE

• This herb can be taken long term for certain conditions, such as chronic asthma, but try to use it only as needed—up to seven days at a time—to minimize the chance of side effects.

• Ephedra interacts with numerous medications, including prescription drugs for heart disease and high blood pressure and various drugs used in hospitals. Be sure to consult your doctor before using the herb.

• Ephedra may be safely combined with many other herbs, including St. John's wort.

• Avoid taking ephedra with caffeine or yohimbine. The combination can cause excessive stimulation.

• If ephedra promotes insomnia, omit your evening dose.

■ Be sure that you buy preparations made from an effective ephedra species, such as *E. sinica*. Many North American species, such as *E. nevadensis* (commonly called Mormon tea, because the first Mormons to reach the arid lands of Utah used this native plant in a piney-tasting tonic), have few active ingredients.

■ Ephedra preparations contain varying amounts of active ingredients called "ephedra alkaloids" that consist primarily of ephedrine. Try to buy preparations with 5.5% to 6.5% alkaloids. A 130 mg dose of ephedra containing 6% alkaloids delivers about 8 mg of ephedrine.

FACTS & TIPS

■ Monitor your pulse and blood pressure when taking ephedra. If your resting heart rate is faster than usual or your blood pressure is high, stop using the herb.

■ Don't take ephedra with over-the-counter cold remedies or with other formulas that have ephedrine or pseudoephedrine. This action will double your dose, raising the likelihood of side effects.

DID YOU KNOW?

Legend has it that Genghis Khan's sentries, threatened with beheading if they fell asleep while on duty, drank a tea brewed from ephedra to stay awake. A cup of ephedra tea delivers about 10 mg of the active ingredient ephedrine.

EVENING PRIMROSE OIL *(Oenothera biennis)*

Native Americans and early settlers in the New World both valued the indigenous evening primrose plant for its healing powers. Today, scientific research is focused largely on the therapeutic effect of the oil derived from the seeds of the plant, which contain a special fat called gamma-linolenic acid (GLA).

COMMON USES

■ Eases rheumatoid arthritis pain.

■ Can minimize symptoms of diabetic nerve damage.

■ Relieves eczema symptoms.

■ Helps treat premenstrual syndrome, endometriosis, and menstrual cramps.

■ Lessens inflammation of acne, rosacea, and muscle strains.

FORMS

■ Capsule

■ Softgel

■ Oil

▼ WHAT IT IS

Called evening primrose because its light yellow flowers open at dusk, this wildflower grows in North America and Europe. The plant and its root have long been used for medicinal purposes—to treat bruises, hemorrhoids, sore throat, and stomachaches.

The use of its seed oil, which contains gamma-linolenic acid (GLA), is relatively recent. GLA is an essential fatty acid that the body converts to hormonelike compounds called prostaglandins, which regulate a number of bodily functions.

Although the body can make GLA from other types of fat you consume, there is no one food that has appreciable amounts of GLA in it. Evening primrose oil provides a concentrated source: 7% to 10% of its fatty acids are in the form of GLA.

There are, however, other sources of GLA. Both borage seed oil and black currant seed oil actually contain higher amounts of GLA (20% to 26% for borage; 14% to 19% for black currant) than evening primrose oil does. But they also have a higher percentage of other fatty acids that may interfere with GLA absorption.

Most of the studies investigating the effects of GLA have used evening primrose oil, and for this reason it is the preferred source of GLA. Still, borage oil may be a good substitute: It is less expensive than evening primrose oil, and a lower dose is required to produce a therapeutic effect.

▼ WHAT IT DOES

The body produces several types of prostaglandins: Some promote inflammation, others control it. The GLA in evening primrose oil is directly converted to important anti-inflammatory prostaglandins, which accounts for most of the supplement's therapeutic effects. In addition, GLA is an important component of cell membranes.

PREVENTION

In people who have diabetes, the GLA in evening primrose oil has been shown to help prevent nerve damage

 ALERT

SIDE EFFECTS

• In studies, about 2% of the participants using evening primrose oil experienced bloating or abdominal upset. However, consuming it with food may lessen this effect.

CAUTION

• Evening primrose oil may increase the risk of seizures in people with schizophrenia who are taking phenothiazine epileptogenic drugs.

• Avoid using evening primrose oil if you are pregnant; its effects on the mother and fetus are unknown.

• **Reminder:** If you have a medical condition, talk to your doctor before taking supplements.

(neuropathy), a common complication of the disease. In a study of people with mild diabetic neuropathy, one year of treatment with evening primrose oil reduced numbness and tingling and other symptoms of the disorder better than a placebo did, suggesting that evening primrose may be of value in reversing neuropathy.

ADDITIONAL BENEFITS
One of the leading uses for evening primrose oil is to treat eczema, an allergic skin condition that may occur if the body has trouble converting fats from food into GLA. Studies of people with eczema indicate that taking evening primrose oil for three to four months can help alleviate itching and reduce the need for topical steroid creams and drugs with unpleasant side effects.

Because of its GLA content, evening primrose oil can be effective for such menstrual disorders as endometriosis, PMS, and menstrual cramps. In particular, the oil blocks the inflammatory prostaglandins that cause menstrual cramps. It also appears to ease the breast tenderness that some women experience just before their periods. Evening primrose oil may also play a role in helping to reverse infertility in some women.

Research studies have found that symptoms of rheumatoid arthritis, an autoimmune disease which is characterized by joint pain and swelling, improve when patients take supplements of evening primrose oil or another source of GLA.

Conditions that involve inflammation, such as rosacea, acne, and muscle strain, can also benefit from evening primrose oil.

▼ HOW TO TAKE IT

DOSAGE
The recommended therapeutic dose for evening primrose oil is generally 1,000 mg three times a day. This supplies 240 mg of GLA a day. To get an equivalent amount of GLA from other sources, you would need to take 1,000 mg of borage oil or 1,500 mg of black currant oil each day.

Evening primrose oil or borage oil can also be applied topically to the fingers to ease the symptoms of poor circulation in Raynaud's disease.

GUIDELINES FOR USE
• Take evening primrose oil or other sources of GLA with meals to enhance the compound's absorption.

Although evening primrose oil comes in liquid form, softgels may be handier to use.

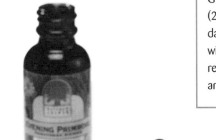

SHOPPING HINTS
■ Many experts recommend buying evening primrose oil that contains a small amount of vitamin E. The fatty acids in evening primrose oil break down quickly; vitamin E slows this process.

LATEST FINDINGS
■ In a study of 60 people with eczema, GLA—the essential fatty acid in evening primrose oil that accounts for its therapeutic benefits—was found to be superior to a placebo in reducing the itching and oozing of the condition. Those in the GLA group took 274 mg twice a day (an amount found in approximately seven 1,000 mg evening primrose capsules) for 12 weeks. Examinations by a dermatologist every four weeks confirmed the gradual improvement of symptoms reported by these patients.

■ A study from the University of Massachusetts Medical Center showed that very high doses of GLA in the form of borage oil (2.4 grams of GLA a day) reduced damage to joint tissue in people with rheumatoid arthritis. As a result, they had less joint pain and swelling.

FEVERFEW *(Tanacetum parthenium)*

Despite its name, feverfew is not a fever reducer but a migraine preventive. Although for centuries this herb was relied on to treat headaches, stomach problems, and menstrual irregularities, feverfew as an herbal remedy virtually disappeared from use until reports calling it a migraine cure began appearing in the late 1970s.

COMMON USES

- Helps prevent or reduce the intensity of migraines.
- May ease menstrual complaints.

FORMS

- Capsule
- Tablet
- Liquid
- Dried herb/Tea

▼ WHAT IT IS

Recently celebrated for its effect on migraines, feverfew (also known as featherfew or febrifuge) belongs to the flower family that includes daisies and sunflowers. With its clear yellow and white blossoms and feathery yellow-green leaves, this herb resembles chamomile and is often mistaken for it.

The plant's leaves are used medicinally, and although the flowers have no health benefits, they do emit a strong aroma. In the Middle Ages, the plant was believed to purify the air and prevent malaria and other life-threatening diseases. Although feverfew probably can't kill germs in the atmosphere, the odor apparently is quite offensive to bees and bugs, so feverfew planted in your garden can act as a natural insect repellent.

▼ WHAT IT DOES

The active compound in feverfew (a chemical called parthenolide) seems to block substances in the body that widen and constrict blood vessels and cause inflammation.

PREVENTION

Though the exact cause of migraines is unknown, some experts think these headaches occur when blood vessels in the head constrict and then rapidly dilate. Such a dramatic change can trigger the release of chemicals stored in platelets (the small blood cells involved in blood clotting) that cause pain and inflammation. Researchers speculate that feverfew prevents the sudden dilation of blood vessels, and so inhibits the release of those chemicals. Though this action makes feverfew a good migraine preventive, the herb cannot relieve a migraine once it occurs.

Word of mouth among people with chronic migraines led to widespread use of feverfew beginning in the

ALERT

SIDE EFFECTS

- Few side effects have been noted, even when feverfew is used over the long term.

- There have been reports of sores and inflammation of the mucous membranes of the mouth, but this reaction seems to be limited to people who chew the fresh leaves (a common practice before feverfew supplements became available).

- Some people experience stomach upset from both the fresh leaves and supplements.

- Skin contact with the plant can cause a rash; anyone who develops a rash after touching feverfew should not use the product internally.

CAUTION

- Pregnant women should avoid feverfew because it may cause contractions of the uterus. Women who are breast-feeding should also not use the herb.

- Feverfew may inhibit blood clotting, so check with your doctor before using this herb if you take anticoagulant drugs (including daily aspirin).

- **Reminder:** If you have a medical condition, talk to your doctor before taking supplements.

1970s. To determine the herb's effectiveness, British researchers recruited migraine sufferers who had already been using feverfew regularly. The researchers then divided them into two sections: One continued to take feverfew, and the other was given a placebo. Those on the placebo pills soon experienced more frequent—and more intense—headaches. But those in the feverfew group had no increase in migraine occurrences.

Another study showed that feverfew reduced the number of migraines by 24% and that even when the headaches did occur, they were much less severe. The results of these and other research studies have led health authorities in Canada and other countries to approve the use of feverfew for migraine prevention.

ADDITIONAL BENEFITS

Feverfew has long been used for menstrual complaints. The herb inhibits the production of prostaglandins, hormonelike substances that can cause pain and inflammation. Because menstrual cramps result from an excess of prostaglandins produced by the lining of the uterus, feverfew may still be suitable for this problem.

The anti-inflammatory action of the herb also led to its use as a treatment for the inflamed, sore joints that occur in rheumatoid arthritis (RA). However, a study of RA patients found no additional benefit from taking feverfew in conjunction with medications that are commonly prescribed for this condition. No studies have been done on how the herb might work alone, or in combination with other herbal treatments for RA.

▼ HOW TO TAKE IT

DOSAGE

For migraines: Take 250 mg a day of either freeze-dried feverfew capsules or a feverfew product standardized to contain at least 0.4% parthenolide.

GUIDELINES FOR USE

• The experience of the migraine sufferers in the British study cited above underscores the importance of taking feverfew daily for an extended time, because stopping the herb may lead to a resumption of headaches.

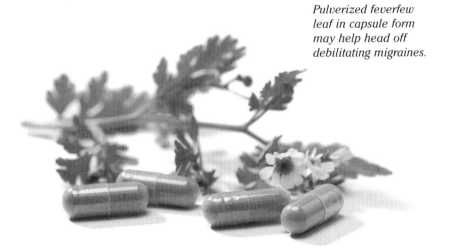

Pulverized feverfew leaf in capsule form may help head off debilitating migraines.

SHOPPING HINTS

■ A study in Great Britain reported that half of the feverfew preparations examined contained virtually none of its active ingredient, parthenolide. Look for tablets and capsules made from the herb *Tanacetum parthenium.* Freeze-dried products are highly rated; standardized products should contain at least 0.4% parthenolide.

CASE HISTORY

A Migraine Preventive

For a while, Nick L. considered the pricey new migraine medications nothing short of wonder drugs because of their amazing ability to stop the dizzying pain of his headaches. But what he really wanted was something that could prevent a migraine from starting. His doctor offered other drugs, but their side effects were troublesome. "Sure, the beta-blockers headed off my migraines," Nick remembers, "but my sex life vanished too." He tried several types, but the result was always the same.

During a trip to London, he saw a shop sign: "Migraine Sufferers— We have feverfew in stock." Though he was skeptical of herbal therapies, he bought a bottle, which sat unopened in his medicine chest for six months. Then he read an article affirming the safety and effectiveness of feverfew and decided to give it a try "From that point on, it was a migraine-free year," he says. "My first since childhood."

FISH OILS

Several years ago scientists noticed a curiously low incidence of heart disease among Greenland Eskimos despite their high-fat diet. The reason? They were eating cold-water fish rich in omega-3 fatty acids. Later studies confirmed the cardioprotective effect of fish oils and uncovered other benefits as well.

COMMON USES

 Help prevent cardiovascular disease; useful for other circulatory conditions as well.

■ Block disease-related inflammatory responses in the body.

■ May lower blood pressure.

FORMS

■ Capsule

■ Softgel

▼ WHAT IT IS

The fat in fish has a form of polyunsaturated fatty acids called omega-3s. These differ from the polyunsaturated fatty acids found in vegetable oils (called omega-6s), and they have different effects on the body. (Fish don't manufacture such fats but get them from the plankton they eat—the colder the water, the more omega-3s the plankton contains.)

The two most potent forms of omega-3s, eicosapentaenoic acid (EPA) and docosahexaenoic acid (DHA), are found in abundance in cold-water fish such as salmon, trout, mackerel, and tuna (including the canned variety). The sources of a third type of omega-3, alpha-linolenic acid (ALA), are certain vegetable oils (such as flaxseed oil) and leafy greens (such as purslane). However, ALA doesn't affect the body in the same way that EPA and DHA do.

▼ WHAT IT DOES

Omega-3s play a key role in a range of vital body processes, from blood pressure and blood clotting to inflammation and immunity. They may be useful for preventing or treating many diseases and disorders.

PREVENTION

Fish oils appear to reduce the risk of heart disease. They do this in several ways. Most importantly, the presence of omega-3s makes platelets in the blood less likely to clump together and form the clots that lead to heart attacks. Next, omega-3s can reduce triglycerides (blood fats that are related to cholesterol) and may lower blood pressure. In addition, recent research has shown that omega-3s strengthen the heart's electrical system, preventing heart-rhythm abnormalities. However, the strongest evidence for the cardiovascular benefits of fish oils comes from studies in which the participants ate fish rather than taking fish oil supplements.

ALERT

SIDE EFFECTS
• Fish oil capsules may cause belching, flatulence, bloating, nausea, and diarrhea.

• Very high doses may result in a slightly fishy body odor.

CAUTION
• Because omega-3 fatty acids inhibit blood clotting, consult a doctor before using fish oil supplements if you have a blood disorder or if you are taking anticoagulants (blood-thinners).

• Individuals with high fasting triglycerides should be careful if they also have high LDL ("bad") cholesterol: Therapeutic doses of fish oils can increase LDL levels.

• People with diabetes should consult their doctor before they start taking fish oil supplements.

• Because omega-3s inhibit blood clotting, avoid taking fish oil supplements two weeks before and one week after surgery .

• **Reminder:** If you have a medical condition, talk to your doctor before taking supplements.

Within the artery walls, omega-3s inhibit inflammation, which is a factor in plaque buildup. As a result, therapeutic doses of fish oils are one of the few successful ways to prevent the reblockage of arteries that commonly occurs after angioplasty, a procedure in which a small balloon is guided through an artery to a blockage and then is inflated to compress plaque, widen the vessel, and improve blood flow to the heart. This effect on blood vessels makes fish oils helpful for Raynaud's disease as well.

ADDITIONAL BENEFITS

Omega-3s are also effective general anti-inflammatories, useful for joint problems, lupus, and psoriasis. Studies indicate that people with rheumatoid arthritis experience less joint swelling and stiffness, and may even be able to manage on lower doses of anti-inflammatory drugs, when they take fish oil supplements. Eating fish probably will not supply enough omega-3 to help rheumatoid arthritis and other inflammatory conditions, so fish oil supplements are recommended.

In a yearlong study of people with Crohn's disease (a painful type of inflammatory bowel disease), 69% of those taking enteric-coated fish oil supplements (about 3 grams of fish oils a day) stayed symptom-free, compared with just 28% of those receiving a placebo. Fish oils may also help ease the inflammation that accompanies menstrual cramps.

In addition, omega-3s may play a role in mental health. Some experts believe there's a correlation between the increasing incidence of depression in the United States and the declining consumption of fish. And a preliminary study suggested that omega-3 fatty acids may reduce the severity of schizophrenia by about 25%.

▼ HOW TO TAKE IT

DOSAGE

For heart disease, Raynaud's disease, lupus, and psoriasis: Take 3,000 mg of fish oils a day.
For rheumatoid arthritis: Take 6,000 mg a day.
For inflammatory bowel disease: Take 5,000 mg a day.

GUIDELINES FOR USE

• Fish oil supplements are not necessary for heart disease prevention or treatment if you eat fish at least twice a week.

• Supplements are recommended for rheumatoid arthritis and other inflammatory conditions.

• Take capsules with meals.

• Supplements may be easier to tolerate if you take them in divided doses. Try 1,000 mg three times a day instead of 3,000 mg in one sitting.

• Some studies have indicated that high doses of fish oils worsen blood sugar control in people with diabetes; others have shown no effect. To be on the safe side, people with diabetes should not take more than 2,000 mg of fish oil supplements a day without the advice of their doctor.

SHOPPING HINTS

■ If you find you can't tolerate one brand of fish oil supplements, try another. Side effects vary from brand to brand.

■ Don't try to save money by buying fish oil supplements in bulk because they can go rancid very quickly. Always store fish oil pills in the refrigerator.

■ Don't buy cod liver oil to get your omega-3s. It contains high amounts of vitamin A and vitamin D, both of which can be toxic in large doses.

LATEST FINDINGS

■ According to a preliminary study from the University of California, Los Angeles, omega-3s may help fight breast cancer and maintain healthy breast tissue. Animal studies also indicate that fewer breast tumors develop when fish oils are part of a healthy diet.

■ Fish oils may help prevent colon cancer. Participants in a recent study who took 4,400 mg of fish oils a day produced much less of one potent carcinogen associated with colon cancer than those on a placebo.

5-HTP

Americans who are suffering from depression, insomnia, migraines, or obesity may have a new supplement to consider: 5-HTP. Unlike its close chemical cousin, the amino acid tryptophan (which was recalled for safety concerns), 5-HTP appears to be safe—and it may be even more effective than tryptophan.

COMMON USES

- Relieves depression.
- Helps overcome insomnia.
- Aids in weight control.
- Treats migraines.
- May ease pain of fibromyalgia.

FORMS

- Capsule
- Tablet

▼ WHAT IT IS

The nutrient 5-HTP, short for 5-hydroxy-tryptophan, is a derivative of the amino acid tryptophan, which is found in such high-protein foods as beef, chicken, fish, and dairy products. The body makes 5-HTP from the tryptophan present in our diets. It's also in the seeds of an African plant (*Griffonia simplicifolia*), which is the source of the 5-HTP supplements sold in health-food stores.

The focus of much recent interest, 5-HTP acts on the brain, helping to elevate mood, promote sleep and weight loss, and relieve migraines, among other uses. Unlike many other supplements (and drugs) that contain substances with molecules too large to pass from the bloodstream into the brain, 5-HTP is small enough to enter the brain. Once there, it is converted into a vital nervous system chemical, or neurotransmitter, called serotonin. Although it affects many parts of the body, serotonin's most important actions take place in the brain, where it influences everything from mood to appetite to sleep.

Because it is closely related to the amino acid tryptophan, 5-HTP remains somewhat controversial. In 1989 the FDA banned tryptophan supplements—which were often sold as L-tryptophan and used for many of the same purposes as 5-HTP—after reports of a fatal illness among those taking it. The illness was later found to be caused by contamination of the supplement during the manufacturing process, not by the tryptophan itself.

In 1994 5-HTP began to be sold in the United States as an over-the-counter alternative to tryptophan. Because 5-HTP is not made in the same way as tryptophan, it avoids the contamination problems of its predecessor. Even though safety concerns have been raised, many experts believe the supplement is safe and effective.

▼ WHAT IT DOES

In recent years 5-HTP has been studied as a treatment for such mood disorders as depression, anxiety, and

ALERT

SIDE EFFECTS
- The generally mild side effects include nausea, constipation, gas, drowsiness, and a reduced sex drive. Nausea usually diminishes within a few days.

CAUTION
- Consult your doctor if you're taking an antidepressant. The combination of 5-HTP with those medications can cause anxiety, confusion, rapid heart rate, sweating, diarrhea, or other adverse reactions.

- Do not drive or do hazardous work until you determine how 5-HTP affects you. It can cause drowsiness in some people.

- **Reminder:** If you have a medical or psychiatric condition, talk to your doctor before taking supplements.

panic attacks because it can boost levels of serotonin in the brain.

Scientists are also investigating whether it may work for a diverse array of additional complaints linked to low serotonin levels, including migraines, fibromyalgia, obesity, eating disorders, PMS, and even violent behavior. Although additional research is needed to determine its effectiveness against many of these conditions, preliminary studies suggest it may be beneficial for some.

MAJOR BENEFITS

For decades, European doctors have been prescribing 5-HTP for the treatment of depression and insomnia. In some cases, it may be more effective, lift depression quicker, and produce fewer side effects than standard antidepressant drugs. In one study, more than half of the patients who suffered from long-term depression and were resistant to all other antidepressants felt better after taking 5-HTP.

The nutrient has also been shown to promote sleep, and to improve the quality of sleep, by increasing the amount of time people spend in two key sleep stages: deep sleep and REM sleep (the dreaming stage). After dreaming longer, those on 5-HTP awaken feeling more rested and refreshed.

ADDITIONAL BENEFITS

Individuals trying to lose weight or suffering from migraines may benefit from 5-HTP. In one study, overweight women who took the supplement ate fewer calories, lost more weight, and were more likely to feel full while on a diet than those given a placebo. It may also be useful in relieving severe headaches, including migraines, reducing not only their frequency, but also their intensity and duration.

The supplement may also work to increase pain tolerance in those with fibromyalgia, a chronic condition marked by aches and fatigue, in part by helping to relieve any underlying depression. In a recent Italian study of 200 fibromyalgia sufferers, those who took 5-HTP along with conventional antidepressants had less pain than those receiving either 5-HTP or the drugs alone. If you're taking antidepressants, don't try 5-HTP without consulting your doctor first: Adverse reactions can occur.

▼ HOW TO TAKE IT

DOSAGE

For depression and most other ailments: Take 50 to 100 mg three times a day.
For migraines: Take up to 100 mg three times a day if necessary.
For insomnia: Take 100 to 200 mg half an hour before bedtime. When using 5-HTP, it is a good idea to begin with a low dose (such as 50 mg) and gradually increase it if needed.

GUIDELINES FOR USE

• To assure rapid absorption, take 5-HTP on an empty stomach.

• Don't use 5-HTP for more than three months without consulting your doctor.

• For weight control, take the supplement 30 minutes before meals.

• Check with your doctor before using 5-HTP with the mood-enhancing herb St. John's wort or adding it to a St. John's wort/ephedra combination (sometimes recommended for weight control). You should also consult your doctor before using 5-HTP with a conventional antidepressant.

SHOPPING HINTS

■ Even though a product is billed as 5-HTP, it may include additional herbs or nutrients that you do not need. Carefully check the ingredient list on the label to make sure you know what you're actually getting.

■ Because 5-HTP is typically sold in 50 mg and 100 mg strengths, you can use the smaller dose to increase your dosage more gradually. This will minimize your risk of suffering side effects.

LATEST FINDINGS

■ Though recent reports of adverse reactions in a few people taking 5-HTP have raised safety concerns, additional study is needed to determine whether these rare reactions are linked to possible contaminants in the supplement. Many experts have found 5-HTP to be safe and effective in large numbers of people.

■ In one recent study, 20 obese patients took either 5-HTP or a placebo for 12 weeks. During the first six weeks, they ate anything they wanted. Over the last six weeks, they restricted their daily diet to 1,200 calories. Those on 5-HTP lost 12 pounds, compared with barely two pounds for the placebo group.

FLANOIDS

What do citrus fruits, grape seed extract, red wine, pine bark extract, apples, and onions have in common? The answer is they're all excellent sources of flavonoids, the colorful plant pigments that help us fight a host of disorders—from heart disease and various types of cancer to vision problems and hay fever.

COMMON USES

■ Reduce the risk of heart disease.

■ May prevent breast, prostate, and other types of cancer.

■ Lessen the chance of age-related vision problems, such as cataracts or macular degeneration.

■ Minimize the symptoms of hay fever and asthma.

■ Fight viral infections.

FORMS

■ Capsule

■ Tablet

■ Powder

■ Liquid

▼ WHAT IT IS

More than 4,000 flavonoids (or bioflavonoids, as they are sometimes called on supplement labels) have been identified, and scientists suspect that there may be many more still to be discovered in nature. Flavonoids give color to fruits, vegetables, and herbs and are found in legumes, grains, and nuts as well.

Flavonoids are also potent antioxidants. Some are even more powerful than vitamin C or vitamin E in neutralizing disease-causing unstable oxygen molecules (free radicals) in the body. So far, however, only a few flavonoids have been studied for their healing potential.

One of these, quercetin (found in onions and apples), also serves as a building block for other flavonoids. Rutin and hesperidin are the most active of the so-called citrus flavonoids,

which, as the name suggests, are present in oranges, grapefruits, tangerines, and other citrus fruits.

Other flavonoids include PCOs (or procyanidolic oligomers; also called proanthocyanidins), anthocyanosides, polyphenols, and genistein. PCOs are plentiful in pine bark and grape seed extracts and in red wine. Anthocyanosides are found in the herb bilberry.

Green tea is the primary source of polyphenols, especially EGCG (epigallocatechin-gallate), which experts believe is possibly the most effective cancer-fighting compound yet discovered. Genistein, found in soy products, has antioxidant properties and can also mimic the effects of estrogen. (For more information, see the profiles on these individual supplements as well.)

▼ WHAT IT DOES

The disease-fighting potential of flavonoids stems from their ability to reduce inflammation, prevent the release of histamine (which causes allergy symptoms such as congestion), fight free radicals, boost immunity, strengthen blood vessels, and increase blood flow, among other actions.

PREVENTION

The flavonoids quercetin and PCOs may protect against heart disease and other circulatory disorders because

ALERT

SIDE EFFECTS

• There are no known toxicities, adverse reactions, or other side effects from flavonoids.

• Flavonoids should be used as complements to—not replacements for—the standard methods for treating cancer, heart diseases, and other serious illnesses.

CAUTION

• **Reminder:** If you have a medical condition, talk to your doctor before taking supplements.

they inhibit bodily changes that can lead to blocked arteries; they also help strengthen blood vessels in various ways.

Studies from Finland and the Netherlands found that people who get plenty of flavonoids, particularly quercetin, have a reduced risk of developing heart disease or having a stroke. In one study, a diet high in flavonoids appeared to cut the chances of dying from heart disease by 50% in women and 23% in men. Another study reported a 75% drop in stroke risk for men who had the highest intake of flavonoids, compared with those who had the lowest.

Polyphenols and quercetin have shown promise as anticancer compounds. Studies found lower rates of stomach, pancreatic, lung, and possibly breast cancer in people with a high intake of these flavonoids. In addition, soy-based genistein may help fight breast cancer and minimize hot flashes by interacting with estrogen receptors in the body. Quercetin also aids the body in using blood sugar and so may be valuable in preventing diabetes. Furthermore, it inhibits the buildup of sorbitol (a type of sugar) in the lens of the eye, a cause of cataracts.

ADDITIONAL BENEFITS
Quercetin may help relieve hay fever, sinusitis, and asthma because it can block allergic reactions to pollen and reduce inflammation in the airways and lungs. This anti-inflammatory action also makes it useful for bug bites, eczema, and related skin conditions, as well as for inflammatory disorders of the joints and muscles, including rheumatoid arthritis, gout, and fibromyalgia.

Because they strengthen blood vessels, PCOs and citrus flavonoids are helpful in repairing varicose veins and hemorrhoids. Rutin and hesperidin play a role in preventing bruising.

▼ HOW TO TAKE IT

DOSAGE
For general health benefits: Buy a flavonoid mixture that contains several types (such as quercetin, rutin, and hesperidin) and follow the dosage instructions on the label.

For allergies, asthma, gout, and insect bites: Take 500 mg quercetin two or three times a day.

GUIDELINES FOR USE
• Grape seed extract and green tea are excellent sources of flavonoids and exert an antioxidant effect as well.

• It's usually a good idea to combine flavonoids with vitamin C to enhance their protective properties.

• Quercetin should be taken 20 minutes before meals; other flavonoids can be taken at any time of the day.

SHOPPING HINTS
■ Mixed preparations of citrus flavonoids are the most widely available and the least expensive supplements of this type. But they are also the least active, often providing a flavonoid content of only 50%. You'll get more value for your dollar by choosing preparations that contain pure rutin, pure hesperidin, or possibly both.

■ Flavonoids are sometimes mixed with vitamin C, and the combination is labeled and sold as vitamin C complex. It's usually less expensive, however, to buy vitamin C and flavonoids separately, which also allows you to vary your dose as needed.

DID YOU KNOW?
Eating an apple a day has always been associated with good health, and a recent study suggests that quercetin may be the magic ingredient. Lung cancer risk fell by 58% in people who ate the most apples (a major source of quercetin) compared with those who ate the fewest apples.

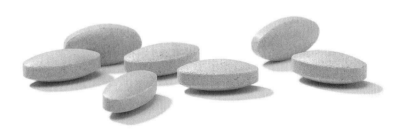

FLAXSEED OIL *(Linum usitatissimum)*

A rich source of healing oil, the common flaxseed has been cultivated for more than 7,000 years. Among the oil's most important uses are the prevention and treatment of cancer, heart disease, and a variety of inflammatory disorders and hormone-related problems. It can also help hair and skin stay healthy.

COMMON USES

■ Helps protect against cancer, heart disease, cataracts, and gallstones.

■ Reduces inflammation associated with gout and lupus.

■ Promotes healthy skin, hair, and nails; treats skin conditions.

■ May be useful for infertility, impotence, and menstrual problems.

■ Aids in treating nerve disorders.

■ Relieves constipation, gallstones, and diverticular disorders.

FORMS

■ Capsule
■ Softgel
■ Oil
■ Powder

▼ WHAT IT IS

It began as a fiber for weaving—and it remains the basis of natural linen fabric. However, the medicinal properties of flaxseeds quickly became legendary. A slender annual that grows up to three feet high and bears blue flowers from February through September, the flax plant was first grown in Europe, then later brought to North America, where it continues to thrive.

Both the oil from the flaxseeds (also known as linseeds) and the seeds are used for therapeutic purposes.

▼ WHAT IT DOES

Flaxseeds are a potent source of essential fatty acids (EFAs)—fats and oils critical for health, which the body cannot make on its own. One EFA, alpha-linolenic acid, is known as an omega-3 fatty acid. Found in fish and flaxseeds, omega-3s have been acclaimed in recent years for protecting against heart disease and for treating many other ailments. Flaxseeds also contain omega-6 fatty acids (in the form of linoleic acid)—the same healthy fats present in many vegetable oils.

In addition, flaxseeds provide substances called lignans, which appear to have beneficial effects on various hormones and may help fight cancer, bacteria, viruses, and fungi. Ounce for ounce, flaxseeds boast up to 800 times the lignans in most other foods.

MAJOR BENEFITS

Essential fatty acids work throughout the body to protect cell membranes—the outer coverings that are gatekeepers for all cells, admitting healthy nutrients and barring damaging substances. That function explains why EFA-rich flaxseed oil has such far-reaching effects.

Flaxseed oil works to lower cholesterol, thereby protecting against heart disease. It may provide benefits as well against angina and high blood pressure. A recent five-year study at Simmons College in Boston indicated that flaxseed oil may be useful in preventing a second heart attack.

 ALERT

SIDE EFFECTS
• Flaxseed oil appears to be very safe. Those using the ground seeds may experience some flatulence initially, but this should soon disappear.

CAUTION
• Some people are allergic to flaxseed. If you experience any difficulty breathing after taking the supplement, seek immediate medical attention.

• Don't ever take flaxseed oil or ground flaxseeds if you have a bowel obstruction of any kind.

• Because of its phytoestrogens, flaxseeds or flaxseed oil should not be used medicinally by pregnant or breast-feeding women.

• **Reminder:** If you have a medical condition, talk to your doctor before taking supplements.

As an anti-inflammatory, flaxseed oil improves the treatment of such conditions as lupus and gout. As a digestive aid, it can help prevent or even dissolve troublesome gallstones. Flaxseed oil also boosts the health of hair and nails and speeds the healing of skin lesions, so it is effective for everything from acne to sunburn.

In addition, flaxseed oil may facilitate the transmission of nerve impulses, making it potentially useful for numbness and tingling, as well as for chronic brain and nerve ailments such as Parkinson's or Alzheimer's disease or nerve damage from diabetes. It may even help fight fatigue.

Crushed flaxseeds are an excellent natural source of fiber. They add bulk to stools, and their oil lubricates the stools, making flaxseeds useful for the relief of constipation, as well as for diverticular complaints.

ADDITIONAL BENEFITS

Flaxseed oil seems to have cancer-fighting properties, though further studies are needed. It may reduce the risk of breast, colon, prostate, and possibly skin cancers. Studies at the University of Toronto found it may also help treat women with early or advanced breast cancer.

Because flaxseeds contain plant-based estrogens (phytoestrogens) that mimic the female sex hormone estrogen, the oil can have beneficial effects on the menstrual cycle, balancing the ratio of estrogen to progesterone. It helps improve uterine function and can therefore treat fertility problems. As an anti-inflammatory, flaxseed oil can reduce menstrual cramps or lessen the pain of fibrocystic breasts.

This oil can promote well-being in men as well. It has shown some promise against male infertility and prostate problems. In some studies, flaxseeds were also found to possess antibacterial, antifungal, and antiviral properties, which may partly explain why flaxseed oil is effective against ailments such as cold sores and shingles.

▼ HOW TO TAKE IT

DOSAGE

Liquid flaxseed oil is the easiest way to get a therapeutic amount, which ranges from 1 teaspoon to 1 tablespoon once or twice a day. To get 1 tablespoon of oil in capsule form, you'll need to swallow about 14 capsules, each containing 1,000 mg of oil.

For flaxseed fiber, mix 1 or 2 tablespoons of ground flaxseeds with a glass of water and drink it up to three times a day; the treatment may take a day or so to act.

GUIDELINES FOR USE

• Always take flaxseed oil with food, which enhances its absorption by the body. You can also mix it into yogurt, cottage cheese, juice, or other foods and drinks.

• Be sure to take ground flaxseed with plenty of water (a large glass per tablespoon) to prevent it from swelling up and blocking your throat or digestive tract.

• Because flax (both the seeds and the oil) can lessen the absorption of other medications, you should separate doses by at least two hours.

SHOPPING HINTS

■ Flaxseed oil spoils fast, so always check the expiration date on the label. To insure freshness, keep it refrigerated. Don't use oil that has a strong or pungent odor.

■ Buy oil that is packaged in an opaque plastic bottle, which filters out oil-spoiling light even better than amber glass. And don't waste your money on "cold-pressed" oil—it's no purer or more healthful than oil processed another way, but it's usually much more costly.

■ Flaxseed oil is also called linseed oil—but never ingest the industrial varieties of linseed oil sold at hardware stores. They are not intended for consumption and may contain toxic additives.

FACTS & TIPS

■ Flaxseed oil has a nutty, buttery taste that many people enjoy. You can add it to salad dressings or sprinkle it over foods; a tablespoon contains just over 100 calories. But do not cook with it, because heat breaks down its nutrients. You can add it to foods after they're cooked, though.

DID YOU KNOW?

A teaspoon of flaxseed oil contains about 2.5 grams of omega-3 fatty acids—more than twice the amount found in the average American's daily diet.

FOLIC ACID

Getting enough of this B vitamin could prevent 50,000 deaths each year from cardiovascular disease. It could also reduce by nearly half the number of babies born with common birth defects and possibly prevent many cancers as well. Yet nine out of ten American adults still take in far too little folic acid.

COMMON USES

■ Protects against birth defects.

■ Reduces the risk of heart disease and stroke.

■ Lowers risk for several cancers.

FORMS

■ Tablet

■ Capsule

■ Powder

■ Liquid

▼ WHAT IT IS

This water-soluble B vitamin, also called folacin or folate, was first identified in the 1940s when it was extracted from spinach. Because the body can't store folic acid very long,, however, you need to replenish your supply daily.

Cooking, or even long storage, can destroy up to half the folic acid in foods, so supplements may be the best way to get an adequate intake of this vital nutrient.

▼ WHAT IT DOES

In the body, folic acid is utilized thousands of times a day to make blood cells, heal wounds, build muscle—in fact, it's necessary for every function that requires cell division.

Folic acid is critical to DNA and RNA formation, and it assures that cells replicate normally. It is especially important in fetal development, helping produce key chemicals for the brain and nervous system.

PREVENTION

Adequate folic acid at conception and for the first three months of pregnancy greatly reduces the risk of serious birth defects, including spina bifida.

This B vitamin also appears to regulate the body's production and use of homocysteine, an amino acid-like substance that at high levels may damage the lining of blood vessels, making them more susceptible to plaque buildup. This makes folic acid an important weapon against heart disease.

In addition, folic acid may help the body to ward off certain cancers, including those of the lungs, cervix, colon, and rectum.

ADDITIONAL BENEFITS

Folic acid may help depression. Because high levels of homocysteine may contribute to this condition, some experts think folic acid (which is often deficient in people who are depressed) may be of value because this nutrient reduces homocysteine levels. Studies also show that taking folic acid improves the effectiveness of antidepressants in people with low folic acid levels.

 ALERT

CAUTION

• Folic acid supplements, even at normal doses, may mask a type of anemia caused by a vitamin B_{12} deficiency. Unchecked, this anemia can cause irreversible nerve damage and dementia. If you take folic acid supplements, be sure to take extra vitamin B_{12} as well.

• Folic acid may reduce the effectiveness of certain anticonvulsant medications. Consult your doctor before taking folic acid supplements if you take medication for a seizure disorder.

• **Reminder:** If you have a medical or psychiatric condition, talk to your doctor before taking supplements.

Folic acid supplements have been useful in treating gout and irritable bowel syndrome as well. Because high homocysteine levels may be a factor in osteoporosis, folic acid may even help keep bones strong.

HOW MUCH YOU NEED

The current adult RDA for folic acid is 400 mcg a day. Supplements are important for older people, who may not get enough of this vitamin in food.

IF YOU GET TOO LITTLE

Though relatively rare, a severe folic acid deficiency can cause a form of anemia (megaloblastic anemia), a sore red tongue, chronic diarrhea, and poor growth (in children). Alcoholics and people who are on certain medications (for cancer or epilepsy) or who have malabsorption diseases (Crohn's, celiac sprue) are susceptible to severe deficiency. Much more common is a low level of folic acid, which causes no symptoms but raises the risk of heart disease or birth defects.

IF YOU GET TOO MUCH

Very large doses–5,000 to 10,000 mcg–offer no benefit and may be dangerous for people with hormone-related cancers, such as those of the breast or prostate. High doses may also cause seizures in those with epilepsy or other seizure disorders.

The National Academy of Sciences suggests an upper daily limit for folic acid of 1,000 mcg for adults.

HOW TO TAKE IT

DOSAGE

For overall good health and the prevention of heart disease: Take 400 to 800 mcg of folic acid a day. *For women who might become pregnant:* Take a total of 800 mcg a day. (Adequate folic acid stores are important because the vitamin plays a role in a baby's development starting with conception.)
For people with depression: Take 800 to 1,200 mcg a day, as part of a vitamin B-complex supplement.

GUIDELINES FOR USE

• Folic acid can be taken at any time of the day, with or without food.

• When taking individual folic acid supplements for any reason, combine it with an additional 1,000 mcg of vitamin B_{12} to prevent a B_{12} deficiency.

OTHER SOURCES

Excellent food sources of folic acid include green vegetables, beans, whole grains, and orange juice. Some refined grain products are now fortified with folic acid.

SHOPPING HINTS

■ Buy a folic acid supplement that also contains vitamin B_{12} (too much of one can mask a deficiency of the other). A combination supplement may be less expensive than buying each vitamin separately.

LATEST FINDINGS

■ For prevention of disease, the best way to get enough folic acid may be through supplements. In a small study, people taking 400 mcg of folic acid a day in pills or in specially fortified foods increased their folic acid level. But those who just ate foods naturally rich in folic acid showed no increase. Scientists speculate that the folic acid found naturally in foods may not be absorbed well enough to have a therapeutic effect.

■ A preliminary study from Oxford University hints that folic acid may play a role in preventing Alzheimer's disease. People with the disease tended to have lower blood levels of folic acid and vitamin B_{12} than healthy people of the same age.

DID YOU KNOW?

You'd need to eat 24 spears of asparagus a day to get the 400 mcg of folic acid recommended for good health.

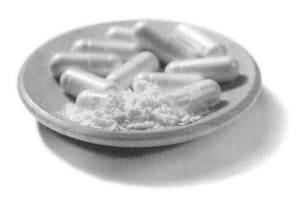

GARLIC *(Allium sativum)*

There was a time when people who wanted to keep their friends wouldn't eat garlic-laced foods and suffer the resulting bad breath. Today, aging baby boomers are more likely to follow the lead of the ancient Egyptians, who worshiped this highly pungent and potent herb for its medicinal and culinary powers.

COMMON USES

- May lower cholesterol levels.
- Reduces blood clotting.
- Fights infections.
- Acts to boost immunity.
- May prevent some cancers.
- May produce a slight drop in blood pressure.
- Combats fungal infections.

FORMS

- Tablet
- Capsule
- Softgel
- Liquid
- Oil
- Powder
- Fresh herb

▼ WHAT IT IS

For thousands of years, garlic has been valued for its therapeutic potential. Once Egyptian pyramid builders took it for strength and endurance; Louis Pasteur investigated its antibacterial properties; and physicians in the two world wars used it to treat battle wounds.

Garlic is related to the onion, scallion, and other plants in the genus *Allium*. The entire plant is odoriferous, but the strongest aroma is concentrated in the bulb, the site of garlic's healing powers and flavor.

Most of garlic's health benefits derive from the more than 100 sulfur compounds it contains. When the bulb is crushed or chewed, alliin, one of the sulfur compounds, becomes allicin, the chemical responsible for garlic's odor and health effects. In turn, some of the allicin is rapidly broken down into other sulfur compounds, such as ajoene, which can also have medicinal properties. Cooking garlic inhibits the formation of allicin and eliminates some of the other therapeutic chemicals.

▼ WHAT IT DOES

Traditionally, garlic has been employed to treat everything from leprosy and parasites to hemorrhoids. Today, researchers are focusing on its potential to reduce the risk of heart disease and cancer.

PREVENTION

The liberal use of garlic in Italy and Spain may partly explain why these countries have such a low incidence of hardening of the arteries (arteriosclerosis). Several studies suggest that garlic can prevent heart disease in various ways. For example, garlic makes platelets (the cells involved in blood clotting) less likely to clump and stick to artery walls, lessening the chance of a heart attack.

There's evidence that the herb dissolves clot-forming proteins, which can affect plaque development. Garlic also lowers blood pressure slightly, mainly because of its ability to widen blood vessels and help blood circulate more freely.

ALERT

SIDE EFFECTS

- Some people develop heartburn, intestinal gas, nausea, and diarrhea when taking garlic, particularly at high doses. Using enteric-coated supplements may reduce such side effects. Skin rashes have also been reported.

CAUTION

- Consult your doctor if you're taking medications to prevent blood clots (anticoagulants, including daily aspirin) or to reduce high blood pressure (antihypertensives). Garlic may intensify the effects of these drugs.

- Avoid garlic supplements before surgery because the herb's anticlotting actions can prolong bleeding.

- **Reminder:** If you have a medical condition, talk to your doctor before taking supplements.

Recent studies examined garlic's effect on cholesterol. Though the results are not clear-cut, most nutritionally oriented doctors think garlic, perhaps in combination with other cholesterol-lowering supplements, is worth a try. The herb may interfere with the metabolism of cholesterol in the liver; as a result, less cholesterol is released into the blood.

ADDITIONAL BENEFITS

Garlic may have anticancer properties. It has been found to be particularly effective in preventing digestive cancers and possibly even breast and prostate cancers. Researchers aren't sure how garlic produces these benefits. Several mechanisms may be involved. First, there's the herb's ability to increase the level of enzymes that can detoxify cancer triggers. Then, it blocks the formation of nitrites linked to stomach cancer. It's also proficient at stimulating the immune system. Garlic's antioxidant properties are important as well.

Garlic is often effective against infectious organisms—viruses, bacteria, and fungi—because allicin can block the enzymes that give the organisms their ability to invade and damage tissues. The herb has also been shown to inhibit the fungi responsible for causing athlete's foot and swimmer's ear.

▼ HOW TO TAKE IT

DOSAGE

Look for supplements that supply 4,000 mcg of allicin potential per pill, approximately the same amount of allicin potential found in one clove of fresh garlic.

For general health or to help high cholesterol: Take a 400 to 600 mg garlic supplement each day.
For colds and flu: Take a 400 to 600 mg garlic supplement four times a day.
For topical benefits: Apply garlic oil two or three times a day. Some skin conditions, including warts and insect bites, may respond to garlic oil or a crushed raw garlic clove applied directly to the affected area.

GUIDELINES FOR USE

• Garlic can be taken indefinitely.

• If you are using the herb for cholesterol problems, have your blood lipid levels checked in three months to see if they have changed; if you've derived no benefits, talk to your doctor about other remedies.

SHOPPING HINTS

■ Most experts believe supplements made from garlic powder are the most effective.

■ Enteric coating prevents garlic breath and allows the supplement to pass through the stomach undigested, which assures the formation of allicin.

■ So-called "deodorized capsules" may effectively remove odor, but manufacturing processes may lessen the garlic's therapeutic effects as well.

LATEST FINDINGS

■ In a recent laboratory study, researchers found that garlic extract was powerful enough to neutralize *Helicobacter pylori,* the bacterium that causes ulcers. The next step is to see if garlic will do the same in the body.

■ Garlic may prevent stiffening of the aorta—the artery that carries blood from the heart to the rest of the body—which occurs naturally with age. In one study, some 200 people took either garlic supplements or a placebo daily for two years. At the study's end, the aortas of the 70-year-olds in the garlic group were as supple as those of the 55-year-olds who didn't take the supplement. A flexible aorta may help reduce age-related organ damage.

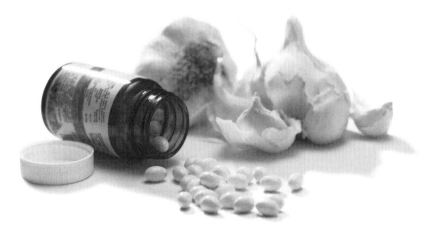

GINGER *(Zingiber officinale)*

From ancient India and China to Greece and Rome, ginger was revered as both a medicinal and culinary spice. Medieval Europeans traced this herb to the Garden of Eden, and it has long been valued by traditional healers. In modern homes and hospitals, it's used to quell nausea and much more.

COMMON USES

- Alleviates nausea and dizziness.
- May relieve pain and inflammation of arthritis.
- Eases muscle aches.
- Relieves allergies.
- Reduces flatulence.

FORMS

- Capsule
- Tablet
- Softgel
- Oil
- Liquid
- Fresh or dried root/Tea
- Crystallized, candied herb

▼ WHAT IT IS

Renowned for its stomach-settling properties, ginger is native to parts of India and China, as well as to Jamaica and other tropical areas. This warm-climate perennial is related to turmeric and marjoram. Its roots are used for culinary and therapeutic purposes.

As a spice, ginger adds a hot and lemony flavor to foods as disparate as roast pork and gingersnap cookies. Medicinally, it continues to play a major role in traditional healing.

▼ WHAT IT DOES

For thousands of years, all around the globe, this pungent spice has been popular as a treatment for digestive problems, ranging from mild indigestion and flatulence to nausea and vomiting. It's also been helpful for relieving colds and arthritis. Modern research into ginger's active ingredients confirms the effectiveness of many of these ancient remedies.

MAJOR BENEFITS

What can you do with a seasick sailor? The answer is: Try ginger. In a Danish study, 40 naval cadets took 1 gram of powdered ginger a day; they were much less likely to break out in a cold sweat and vomit (classic symptoms of being seasick) than 39 others who took a placebo.

Because ginger works primarily in the digestive tract, boosting digestive fluids and neutralizing acids, it may be a good medical alternative to antinausea drugs that can affect the central nervous system and cause grogginess. Clinical studies of women undergoing exploratory surgery (laparoscopy) or major gynecological surgery show that taking 1 gram of ginger before an operation can significantly reduce postoperative nausea and vomiting, a common side effect of anesthetics and other medications given in surgery.

Ginger also appears to counter the nausea created by chemotherapy, though it's best to take it with food to minimize any stomach irritation.

 ALERT

SIDE EFFECTS

- Ginger is very safe for a broad range of complaints; occasional heartburn has been the only documented side effect.

CAUTION

- Consult your doctor if unusual or unexpected bleeding develops while taking ginger.

- Ginger may relieve morning sickness during the first two months of pregnancy (up to 250 mg four times a day). But longer use or higher doses should be taken only under a doctor's supervision.

- Chemotherapy patients should not take ginger on an empty stomach because it can irritate the stomach lining.

- **Reminder:** If you have a medical condition, talk to your doctor before taking supplements.

Ginger's antinausea effects make it useful for reducing dizziness (common in older patients), as well as for treating morning sickness. For years, ginger has been a staple of folk medicine, serving primarily as a digestive aid.

Ginger supplements (or fresh pulp mixed with lime juice) are also a fine remedy for flatulence.

ADDITIONAL BENEFITS
Ginger's anti-inflammatory and pain-relieving properties may help relieve the muscle aches and chronic pain associated with arthritis and other conditions. In a study of seven women with rheumatoid arthritis (an autoimmune disease characterized by severe inflammation), just 5 to 50 grams of fresh ginger or capsules containing up to 1 gram of powdered ginger lessened joint pain and inflammation.

Its anti-inflammatory properties suggest that ginger may ease bronchial constriction due to allergies or colds.

▼ HOW TO TAKE IT

DOSAGE
To prevent motion sickness, dizziness, and nausea; reduce flatulence; and relieve chronic pain or rheumatoid arthritis: Take ginger up to three times a day, or every four hours as needed. The usual dose is 100 to 200 mg of the standardized extract in pill form; 1 or 2 grams of fresh powdered ginger; or a ½-inch slice of fresh ginger root.

Other preparations, including ginger tea (available in tea bags, or use ½ teaspoon of grated ginger root per cup of very hot water) or natural ginger ale (containing real ginger), can be used several times a day for similar purposes and for arthritis and pain relief. On trips, try crystallized ginger candy: A 1-inch square, about ¼-inch thick, contains about 500 mg of ginger.

For aching muscles: Rub several drops of ginger oil, mixed with ½ ounce of almond oil or another neutral oil, on the sore areas.
For allergy relief: Drink up to four cups of ginger tea a day as needed to reduce symptoms.

GUIDELINES FOR USE
• Take ginger capsules with fluid. If you are trying to prevent motion sickness, have ginger three to four hours before your departure, and then take it every four hours as needed, up to four times a day.

• For postoperative nausea, begin taking ginger the day before your operation—but only under a doctor's supervision. Medical oversight is needed because ginger has the ability to increase bleeding under certain circumstances.

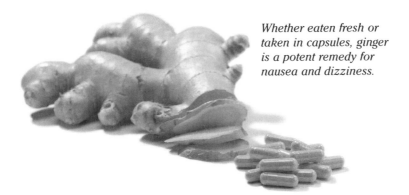

Whether eaten fresh or taken in capsules, ginger is a potent remedy for nausea and dizziness.

SHOPPING HINTS
■ Buy ginger supplements standardized to contain "pungent compounds." These consist of gingerols and shogaols—the active ingredients that give ginger its healing properties.

■ Look for natural ginger ales made from real ginger: An 8-ounce glass contains about a gram of ginger. Most widely distributed commercial ginger ales have only tiny amounts of ginger or ginger flavoring, which have no therapeutic benefits at all.

FACTS & TIPS
■ The ancient Greeks so prized ginger for digestion that they mixed it into their bread. Thus was born the first gingerbread.

■ American colonists brewed a stomach-soothing remedy called ginger beer—a forerunner of today's ginger ale.

■ For colds or flu, many folk healers recommend chewing fresh ginger, drinking ginger tea, or squeezing juice from ginger root into a spoonful of honey. All may help ease the aches and chest tightness associated with these infections.

DID YOU KNOW?
A cup of ginger tea contains the equivalent of about 250 mg of the powdered herb. A heavily spiced Chinese or Indian ginger dish has about twice that amount.

GINKGO BILOBA *(Ginkgo biloba)*

This popular herbal medicine is derived from one of the oldest species of tree on earth, and today it is widely marketed as a general memory booster. Ginkgo biloba does seem to help with age-related memory loss, but whether this high profile herb is a universal "smart pill" that's meant for everyone remains to be seen.

COMMON USES

■ Slows progression of Alzheimer's; sharpens memory and concentration.

■ Lessens depression and anxiety.

■ Alleviates coldness in the extremities and painful leg cramps.

■ Helps headaches, ringing in the ears (tinnitus), and dizziness.

■ May restore impotent men's erections.

FORMS

■ Tablet

■ Capsule

■ Softgel

■ Powder

■ Liquid

▼ WHAT IT IS

The medicinal form of the herb is extracted from the fan-shaped leaves of the ancient ginkgo biloba tree, a species that has survived in China for more than 200 million years. (The leaves are double- or bi-lobed; hence the name "biloba.")

A concentrated form of the herb called ginkgo biloba extract (GBE) is used to make the dietary supplement that is sold in stores all over the United States today. Commonly called ginkgo, GBE is obtained by drying and milling the plant's leaves and then extracting the active ingredients in a mixture of acetone and water.

▼ WHAT IT DOES

Ginkgo may have beneficial effects on both the circulatory and the central nervous systems. It increases blood flow to the brain and to the arms and legs by regulating the tone and elasticity of blood vessels, from the largest arteries to the tiniest capillaries. It also acts like aspirin by helping to reduce the "stickiness" of the blood, thereby lowering the risk of blood clots.

Ginkgo appears to have antioxidant properties as well, mopping up the damaging compounds known as free radicals and aiding in the maintenance of healthy blood cells. And some researchers report that it enhances the nervous system by promoting the delivery of additional oxygen and blood sugar (glucose) to nerve cells.

PREVENTION

Interest now centers on ginkgo's possible role as a preventive for age-related memory loss. Unfortunately, there's little scientific evidence that ginkgo will make most people better able to focus or remember. So far, it is those already suffering from diminished blood flow to the brain—not healthy volunteers—who have benefited most from taking the herb.

Current research is trying to determine whether ginkgo's ability to help prevent blood clots may stave off heart attacks or strokes.

 ALERT

SIDE EFFECTS

• Rarely, ginkgo may cause irritability, restlessness, diarrhea, nausea, or vomiting; a headache may occur initially too. These effects are usually transient; if they persist, reduce the dosage or stop taking the herb.

CAUTION

• Doses above 240 mg a day can cause disorientation and other problems.

• Don't use unprocessed ginkgo leaves in any form, including teas; they contain potent chemicals (allergens) that can trigger allergic reactions. Stick with standardized extracts (GBE) because allergens are removed.

• People scheduled for surgery who take anticoagulants (including aspirin) or who suffer from a clotting disorder should consult a doctor before taking ginkgo because it slows the rate at which blood clots.

• **Reminder:** If you have a medical or psychiatric condition, talk to your doctor before taking supplements.

MAJOR BENEFITS

The fact that ginkgo aids blood flow to the brain—thus increasing oxygen—is of particular relevance to older people, whose arteries may have narrowed with cholesterol buildup or other conditions. Diminished blood flow has been linked to Alzheimer's and memory loss, as well as to anxiety, headaches, depression, confusion, ringing in the ears, and dizziness. All may be helped by ginkgo.

ADDITIONAL BENEFITS

Ginkgo also promotes blood flow to the arms and legs, making it useful for reducing the pain, cramping, and weakness caused by narrowed arteries in the leg, a disorder called intermittent claudication. There are indications that the herb may improve circulation to the extremities in those with Raynaud's disease, or help victims of scleroderma, an uncommon autoimmune disorder.

In addition, by increasing blood flow to the nerve-rich fibers of the eyes and ears, some studies suggest ginkgo may be of value in treating macular degeneration or diabetes-related eye disease (both leading causes of blindness), as well as some types of hearing loss.

Ongoing studies are assessing the possible effectiveness of ginkgo in speeding up recovery from certain strokes and head injuries, as well as in treating conditions that may be related to circulatory or nervous system impairment,

including impotence, multiple sclerosis, and nerve damage that is frequently associated with diabetes. Traditional Chinese healers have long used ginkgo for asthma, because the herb appears to alleviate wheezing as well as other respiratory complaints.

▼ HOW TO TAKE IT

DOSAGE

Always take supplements that contain ginkgo biloba extract—or GBE—the concentrated form of the herb.

As a general memory booster and for poor circulation: Take 120 mg of GBE daily, divided into two or three doses, or 1 teaspoon liquid extract three times a day.
For Alzheimer's disease, depression, ringing in the ears, dizziness, impotence, or other conditions caused by insufficient blood flow to the brain: Take up to 240 mg a day.

GUIDELINES FOR USE

• It commonly takes four to six weeks, and in some cases up to 12 weeks, to notice the herb's effects.

• You can take ginkgo biloba with or without food.

• Ginkgo biloba is generally considered safe for long-term use when it's taken in recommended dosages.

SHOPPING HINTS

■ Be certain that you buy preparations with ginkgo biloba extract to ensure you're getting a standardized amount of the active ingredients. GBE supplements should contain at least 24% flavone glycosides (organic substances responsible for the herb's antioxidant and anticlotting properties) and 6% terpene lactones (primarily chemicals called ginkgolides and bilobalides, which improve blood flow and are thought to protect the nerves).

LATEST FINDINGS

■ A yearlong study published in the *Journal of the American Medical Association* evaluated 202 patients with dementia, most of whom also had Alzheimer's disease. Patients who took 120 mg of ginkgo biloba extract a day were more likely to stabilize or improve their mental and social functions, compared with those given a placebo. The effects were modest and of limited duration.

DID YOU KNOW?

Ginkgo trees have two "sexes"—male and female. The nuts from the female tree are still valued in China and Japan as a culinary delicacy with healing properties.

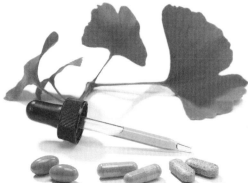

Derived from ginkgo biloba leaves, the herb is effective in either pill or liquid form.

GINSENG (PANAX) *(Panax ginseng)*

A wildly popular herb in the United States and Europe, ginseng is added to everything from fruit juices to vitamin supplements. Though most of these products actually contain very little ginseng and are typically ineffective, supplements made with quality ginseng do indeed exert a variety of protective effects on the body.

COMMON USES

- Combats the damaging physical effects of stress.
- May treat impotence and infertility in men.
- Boosts energy.

FORMS

- Tablet
- Capsule
- Softgel
- Powder
- Liquid/Tincture
- Dried herb/Tea

▼ WHAT IT IS

Panax ginseng (also commonly called Asian, Chinese, or Korean ginseng) has been used in Chinese medicine for thousands of years to enhance longevity and the quality of life. *Panax ginseng* is the most widely available and extensively studied form of this herb. Another species, *Panax quinquefolius,* or American ginseng, is grown mainly in the Midwest and exported to China.

The medicinal part of the plant is its slow-growing root, which is harvested after four to six years, when its overall ginsenoside content—the main active ingredient in ginseng—is at its peak. There are 13 different ginsenosides in all. Panax ginseng also contains panaxans, substances that can lower blood sugar, and polysaccharides, complex sugar molecules that enhance the immune system.

"White" ginseng is simply the dried root; "red" ginseng has been steamed and dried.

▼ WHAT IT DOES

The primary health benefits of Panax ginseng derive from its immune-stimulating and antioxidant properties, as well as from its ability to protect the body against the effects of stress.

PREVENTION

Ginseng may help the body combat a variety of illnesses. It stimulates the production of specialized immune cells called "killer T cells," which destroy harmful viruses and bacteria.

Studies have also indicated that the herb may inhibit the growth of certain cancer cells. A large Korean study found that the risk of developing cancer in people who took ginseng was half that of those who did not take it. Interestingly, although ginseng powders and tinctures were shown to have cancer-preventive effects, eating fresh ginseng root or drinking ginseng juice or tea did not lower the cancer risk.

  ALERT

SIDE EFFECTS
- At the doses recommended here, ginseng is unlikely to cause any noticeable side effects.

- Higher doses, however, may cause nervousness, insomnia, headache, and stomach upset; if you have any of these problems, reduce your dose.

- Some women report increased menstrual bleeding or breast tenderness with high doses of ginseng. If this occurs, reduce the dose or stop using it.

CAUTION
- Don't take Panax ginseng if you have uncontrolled high blood pressure or a heart rhythm irregularity, or if you are pregnant.

- Don't use Panax ginseng if you take MAO inhibitor drugs, diabetes medication, diuretics, methylphenidate (Ritalin), high blood pressure drugs, or oral corticosteroids.

- **Reminder:** If you have a medical condition, talk to your doctor before taking supplements.

ADDITIONAL BENEFITS

Ginseng may benefit people who are feeling fatigued and overstressed and those recovering from a long illness. The herb has been shown to balance the release of stress hormones in the body and support the organs that produce these hormones, namely the pituitary gland and hypothalamus in the brain and the adrenal glands, located on top of the kidneys. Ginseng may also enhance the production of endorphins, "feel-good" chemicals produced by the brain.

Many long-distance runners and bodybuilders take ginseng to heighten physical endurance. Some nutritionally oriented doctors and herbalists believe that ginseng is able to delay fatigue because it enables the exercising muscles to use energy more efficiently. There is research, however, that contradicts this hypothesis.

Though the way it works is not clear, ginseng may be helpful for impotence. Some of its active ingredients appear to affect smooth muscle tissue and improve erectile function. Men with fertility problems may benefit from ginseng as well because animal studies indicate it increases testosterone levels and sperm production.

▼ HOW TO TAKE IT

DOSAGE
Select a product that is standardized to contain at least 7% ginsenosides.

For general health and combating fatigue: Take 100 to 250 mg Panax ginseng in capsules or 1 teaspoon liquid extract once or twice a day.
To support the body in times of stress or during recovery from an illness: Take 100 to 250 mg or 1 teaspoon liquid extract twice a day.
For male impotence and infertility: Take 100 to 250 mg or 1 teaspoon liquid extract twice a day.

GUIDELINES FOR USE
• Start at the lower end of the dosage range and increase your intake gradually until you begin to feel better.

• Some experts recommend that you stop taking ginseng for a week every two or three weeks and then resume your regular dose. In some cases, ginseng may be rotated with other immune-stimulating herbs, such as astragalus or Siberian ginseng.

• The combination of ginseng and caffeine may intensify any side effects, so cut back on (or avoid) caffeine.

SHOPPING HINTS
■ Read labels carefully to be sure you're getting *Panax ginseng.* Other kinds, such as American ginseng (*Panax quinquefolius*) and Siberian ginseng (*Eleutherococcus senticosus*), produce different effects.

■ Vials of ginseng elixir sold at convenience stores have become popular energy tonics, especially among young kids and teens. They often contain little (if any) ginseng, however, and may have a high alcohol content.

LATEST FINDINGS
■ People with type 2, or non-insulin-dependent, diabetes may benefit from ginseng. In one study, participants with diabetes who took 100 or 200 mg of ginseng a day had lower blood sugar levels than those given a placebo. Always consult a doctor before taking ginseng with a diabetes medicine, however.

DID YOU KNOW?
The name "ginseng" is derived from the ancient Chinese word *jen shen,* which literally means "man root." This is because the ginseng root (shown at left) often resembles the shape of the human body.

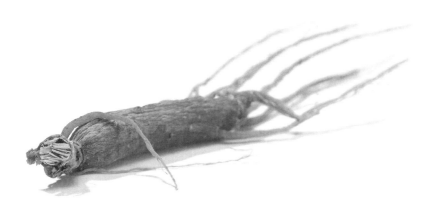

GLUCOSAMINE

This promising and popular arthritis fighter helps build cartilage, which provides cushioning at the tips of the bones. It also protects and strengthens the joints as it relieves the pain and stiffness that often accompany this degenerative condition. Although your body produces some glucosamine, a supplement is more effective.

COMMON USES

■ Relieves pain, stiffness, and swelling due to osteoarthritis or rheumatoid arthritis, which affect the knees, fingers, and other joints.

■ Helps reduce arthritic back and neck pain.

■ May speed the healing of sprains and strengthen joints, preventing future injury.

FORMS

■ Capsule

■ Tablet

■ Powder

▼ WHAT IT IS

Scientists have long known that the body manufactures a small amount of glucosamine (pronounced glue-KOSE-a-mean), a fairly simple molecule that contains the sugar glucose. It's found in relatively high concentrations in the joints and connective tissues, where the body uses it to form the larger molecules necessary for cartilage repair and maintenance.

In recent years, glucosamine has become available as a nutritional supplement. Various forms are sold, including glucosamine sulfate and N-acetyl-glucosamine (NAG). Glucosamine sulfate is the preferred form for arthritis: It is readily used by the body (90% to 98% is absorbed through the intestine) and appears to be very effective for this condition.

▼ WHAT IT DOES

Though some experts hail glucosamine as an arthritis cure, no one supplement can claim that title. It does, however, provide significant relief from pain and inflammation for about half of arthritis sufferers—especially those with the common age-related form known as osteoarthritis. It can also help people with rheumatoid arthritis and other types of joint injuries, and it offers additional benefits as well.

MAJOR BENEFITS

Approved for the treatment of arthritis in at least 70 countries around the world, glucosamine has been shown to ease pain and inflammation, increase range of motion, and help repair aging and damaged joints in the knees, hips, spine, and hands.

Recent studies show that glucosamine may be even more effective for relieving pain and inflammation than aspirin, ibuprofen, and other nonsteroidal anti-inflammatory drugs (NSAIDs)—and without the side effects of NSAIDs. While NSAIDs, commonly taken by arthritis sufferers, mask arthritis pain, they do little to combat the progression of the disease—and may even make it worse by impairing the body's ability to build cartilage.

In contrast, glucosamine helps make cartilage and may repair damaged joints. Though it can't do much for

ALERT

SIDE EFFECTS
• Glucosamine is virtually free of side effects, although gastrointestinal effects, such as heartburn or nausea, occasionally occur. Drowsiness, headache, and rash have also been reported.

CAUTION
• Glucosamine may interact with certain diuretic drugs, necessitating higher doses of the diuretic. Consult your doctor for guidance.

• **Reminder:** If you have a medical condition, talk to your doctor before taking supplements.

people with advanced arthritis, when cartilage has completely worn away, it may benefit the millions of people with mild to moderately severe symptoms.

ADDITIONAL BENEFITS

As a joint strengthener, glucosamine may be useful for the prevention of arthritis and many forms of age-related degenerative joint disease. It may also help to speed the healing of acute joint injuries, such as a badly sprained ankle or finger.

In addition to aiding joints and connective tissues, glucosamine promotes a healthy lining in the digestive tract and may be beneficial in treating ailments such as irritable bowel syndrome. It is included in various "intestinal health" preparations sold in health-food stores, usually in the form of NAG (N-acetyl-glucosamine), which tends to act specifically on the intestinal lining.

▼ HOW TO TAKE IT

DOSAGE

The standard dosage for arthritis and other conditions is 500 mg glucosamine sulfate three times a day. For convenience, the entire dose of 1,500 mg can be taken once daily in either pill or powder form. (Packets containing a daily dose of powdered glucosamine are convenient; mix into a glass of water).

This amount (1,500 mg) has been shown to be safe for all individuals and effective for most. People weighing more than 200 pounds or taking diuretics may need higher daily doses (about 900 mg per 100 pounds of body weight); talk to your doctor about determining an appropriate dosage.

GUIDELINES FOR USE

• Glucosamine is typically taken long term and appears to be very safe. It may not bring relief as quickly as pain relievers or anti-inflammatories (it usually works in two to eight weeks), but its benefits are far greater and longer-lasting when it's used over an extended period of time.

• Take glucosamine with meals. Food will help to minimize the chance of digestive upset.

• Glucosamine's anti-arthritis effects may be enhanced by using it along with another supplement, such as chondroitin sulfate (a related cartilage-building compound), niacinamide (a form of the B vitamin niacin), or S-adenosylmethionine (SAMe), a form of the amino acid methionine. Other supplements that are sometimes taken along with glucosamine for the relief of arthritis include boswellia, a tree extract from India; sea cucumber, an ancient Chinese remedy; and the topical pain reliever cayenne cream.

• No adverse reactions have been reported when glucosamine is used with prescription or over-the-counter drugs or with other supplements.

FACTS & TIPS

■ Supplements are actually the best source of extra glucosamine because dietary sources of the nutrient are quite obscure. Items that are relatively rich in glucosamine include the shells of shrimp, crabs, and oysters.

■ Scientists in San Diego believe that oral administration of glucosamine for a few days immediately following surgery may help speed healing. It may also reduce surgical scarring and the complications it can cause, suggesting another possible use for this supplement.

LATEST FINDINGS

■ A study conducted in China at the Beijing Union Medical College Hospital, involving 178 patients with osteoarthritis of the knee, showed that 1,500 mg of glucosamine sulfate taken daily was just as effective in reducing the symptoms of the disease as 1,200 mg of ibuprofen—and was significantly better tolerated by the patients.

DID YOU KNOW?

Older dogs that have trouble getting around because of stiff joints may benefit from glucosamine sulfate. It has been shown to be as safe and effective for canines as it is for their masters.

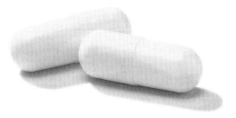

GOLDENSEAL *(Hydrastis canadensis)*

For centuries, Cherokee, Iroquois, and other Native American tribes have valued the root of the goldenseal plant as a remedy for everything from insect bites and bloating to eye infections and stomachaches. Today, this versatile herb is officially recognized as a medicine in eleven countries—though not yet in the United States.

COMMON USES

- Promotes healing of canker sores and cold sores.
- Helps destroy the different viruses that cause warts.
- Bolsters the immune system.
- Calms a nauseated stomach.
- May help urinary tract infections.
- Treats eye infections.

FORMS

- Capsule
- Softgel
- Liquid
- Dried herb/Tea
- Ointment/Cream

▼ WHAT IT IS

The dried root of this perennial herb has long been used to soothe inflamed or infected mucous membranes. Today, it is appreciated for its ability to help the body fight infection.

The plant was first called goldenseal in the nineteenth century, deriving its name from the rich yellow of the root and the small cuplike scars found there. These scars, which appear on the previous year's root growth, resemble the wax seals that were once used to close envelopes—hence the name "goldenseal."

Related to the buttercup, goldenseal is native to North America and once grew wild from Vermont to Arkansas. As interest in the herb's medicinal properties grew, however, the plant was extensively harvested. Currently, most of the goldenseal on the market is commercially cultivated in Oregon and Washington.

The key medicinal compounds in goldenseal are the alkaloids berberine and hydrastine. Berberine is also responsible for the root's rich yellow color—so vibrant, in fact, that Native Americans and early settlers utilized goldenseal as a dye as well as a medicinal herb. Because the alkaloids have a bitter taste, goldenseal tea often includes other herbs, or it can be mixed with a sweetener such as honey.

▼ WHAT IT DOES

The primary benefit of goldenseal is its overall effect on immunity. Not only does it increase the immune system's production of germ-fighting compounds, this herb can combat both bacteria and viruses directly.

PREVENTION
Taking goldenseal at the first sign of a cold or the flu may prevent the illness from developing fully—or at least greatly minimize the symptoms—by enhancing the activity of virus-fighting white blood cells.

ADDITIONAL BENEFITS
Goldenseal fights bacteria, making it useful for mild urinary tract infections (if you begin taking it early enough)

 ALERT

SIDE EFFECTS
- When taken at recommended doses and for suggested (limited) lengths of time, goldenseal has few side effects.

- Very high doses may irritate the mucous membranes of the mouth and cause diarrhea, nausea, respiratory problems, and even seizures and other serious complications. Seek medical attention if high doses are taken.

CAUTION
- Goldenseal should not be used by pregnant women or people with heart disease, high blood pressure, diabetes, or glaucoma.

- **Reminder:** If you have a medical condition, talk to your doctor before taking supplements.

and sinus infections. It may also help soothe nausea and vomiting, by stimulating digestive secretions and working to destroy the bacteria that may be causing the symptoms.

As one of several herbs that stimulate the immune system—others include echinacea, pau d'arco, and astragalus—goldenseal may play a role in relieving the symptoms of chronic fatigue syndrome, a disabling disorder that may be partially caused by a weakened immune system. It also helps to fight cold sores and shingles (both caused by the herpes virus). Use it for no more than a week or two at a time.

Applied topically, goldenseal tincture is beneficial for canker sores and warts. The liquid extract promotes healing of the sores and directly fights the human papilloma viruses that cause warts.

Once cooled and strained, goldenseal tea can be used as an eyewash to relieve eye infections such as conjunctivitis. Be sure to prepare a fresh batch daily and store it in a sterile container, so the tea won't get contaminated.

▼ HOW TO TAKE IT

DOSAGE
For colds, flu, and other respiratory infections: As soon as you begin to feel sick, take 125 mg of goldenseal (in combination with 200 mg of echinacea) five times a day for five days.

For urinary tract infections: Drink several cups of freshly brewed goldenseal tea daily.

For nausea and vomiting: Take 125 mg every four hours as needed.

For chronic fatigue syndrome: Use 125 mg twice a day in rotation with other immune-stimulating herbs.

For cold sores: Take 125 mg of goldenseal with 200 mg echinacea four times a day.

For shingles: Take 125 mg of goldenseal with 200 mg echinacea four times a day.

For canker sores and warts: Apply goldenseal liquid extract directly to the sores three times a day.

For eye infections: Use 1 teaspoon dried herb per pint of hot water. Steep, finely strain, cool, and apply as an eyewash three times a day; make a new solution every day.

GUIDELINES FOR USE
• Take goldenseal with meals.

• Use goldenseal only when you feel that you're coming down with a cold, the flu, or some other illness, and just for the duration of the illness.

• As a general rule, don't use goldenseal for more than three weeks at a time. And wait two weeks, at least, before taking it again.

SHOPPING HINTS

■ When buying goldenseal, look for extracts standardized to contain 8% to 10% alkaloids or 5% hydrastine.

CASE HISTORY

Go for the Gold
Alexa K. always reacted badly to antibiotics. Although she knew she needed them for her sinus infections, the side effects (dizziness, nausea, diarrhea) often made the drugs worse than the illness.

When an herbalist told her to try goldenseal extract, her doctor was skeptical. "Look," he said, "try the goldenseal, but keep my prescription handy. If you don't feel better, you can always get it filled."

Alexa took the goldenseal, and in a few days her sinus infection was gone—without a single side effect. Now goldenseal is a part of her sinus first-aid kit. At the first sign of an infection, she starts taking it, along with the immune stimulator echinacea.

Although antibiotics are sometimes necessary, in the last few years Alexa has often been able to avoid them. "Those miserable side effects are history!" she happily reports.

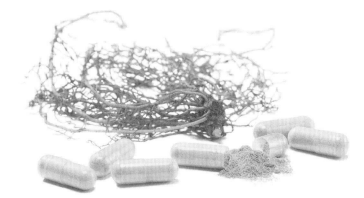

The root of the goldenseal plant is dried and then ground to a fine powder for use in supplements.

97

GOTU KOLA *(Centella asiatica)*

Because this herb from India has long been a favorite food of elephants, notoriously long-lived animals, many people associate its use with longevity. Even though scientific research hasn't shown that this plant can extend your life, studies have found that gotu kola does provide many other important health benefits.

COMMON USES

- Treats burns and wounds.
- Builds connective tissue.
- Strengthens veins.
- Improves memory.

FORMS

- Capsule
- Tablet
- Liquid
- Powder
- Dried herb/Tea

▼ WHAT IT IS

The medicinal use of gotu kola has its roots in India, where the herb continues to be part of the ancient healing tradition called Ayurveda. Word of its therapeutic benefits for skin disorders gradually spread throughout Asia and Europe. In fact, gotu kola has been prescribed in France since the 1880s to treat burns and other wounds.

A red-flowered plant that thrives in hot, swampy areas, gotu kola grows naturally in India, Sri Lanka, Madagascar, middle and southern Africa, Australia, China, and the southern United States.

The appearance of this slender, creeping perennial changes depending on whether it's growing in water (broad, fan-shaped leaves) or on dry land (small, thin leaves). The plant's leaf is most commonly used medicinally.

▼ WHAT IT DOES

Whether taken internally or applied externally as a compress, gotu kola has many beneficial effects. The herb's workhorse substances are chemicals called triterpenes (especially asiaticoside), which appear to enhance the formation of collagen in bones, cartilage, and connective tissue. In addition, they promote healthy blood vessels and help produce neurotransmitters, the chemical messengers in the brain.

MAJOR BENEFITS

Gotu kola's singular effect on connective tissue—promoting its healthy development and inhibiting the formation of hardened areas—makes this herb potentially important for treating many skin conditions. It can be therapeutic for burns, keloids (overgrown scar tissue), and wounds (including surgical incisions and skin ulcers).

Gotu kola also seems to strengthen cells in the walls of blood vessels, improving blood flow and making it valuable for the treatment of varicose veins. Research results have been impressive. In more than a dozen studies observing gotu kola's effect on veins (which are surrounded by supportive connective-tissue sheaths),

 ALERT

SIDE EFFECTS

- Taking gotu kola orally or using a topical preparation generally does not cause problems.

- Skin rash (dermatitis), sensitivity to sunlight, and headaches are rare side effects. If you experience these symptoms, reduce the dosage or stop using the herb.

CAUTION

- Pregnant women or those who are trying to conceive should not use gotu kola.

- **Reminder:** If you have a medical condition, talk to your doctor before taking supplements.

about 80% of patients with varicose veins and similar problems showed substantial improvement.

Other studies indicate that applying gotu kola topically to psoriasis lesions may aid healing as well.

ADDITIONAL BENEFITS

Gotu kola has been used to increase mental acuity for thousands of years. Current research supports a role for this herb in boosting memory, improving learning capabilities, and possibly reversing some of the memory loss associated with Alzheimer's disease.

In one study, 30 developmentally disabled children were found to have significantly better concentration and attention levels after taking gotu kola for 12 weeks than they did at the start of the study. Preliminary findings reveal that animals given gotu kola for two weeks were able to learn and retain new behaviors much better than animals not on the herb.

▼ HOW TO TAKE IT

DOSAGE

To treat varicose veins: Take 40 to 60 mg of the standardized extract or 400 to 600 mg dried whole herb three times a day.

For burns: Apply gotu kola liquid extract or a strong (cooled) gotu kola tea (see below) to the burn twice a day

To improve memory or help slow the progress of Alzheimer's disease: Take 40 to 60 mg of the standardized extract or 400 to 600 mg of the dried whole herb three times a day.

GUIDELINES FOR USE

• You can use both the oral and topical preparations of the herb over the same period of time.

• Internally, gotu kola is usually taken in the form of a tablet or capsule, with or without meals.

• Topically, a gotu kola tea or a liquid extract can be applied externally to the skin for psoriasis, burns, wounds, incisions, or scars. To apply gotu kola topically, soak a compress in tea or in 1 to 2 teaspoons of liquid extract and apply it directly to problem areas. Start with a relatively weak solution and increase the strength as needed.

• To brew gotu kola tea, steep 1 or 2 teaspoons of dried leaf in a cup of very hot water for 10 to 15 minutes.

• To make a paste to apply to patches of skin affected by psoriasis: Break open capsules and mix 2 teaspoons of dried gotu kola powder in a small amount of water.

SHOPPING HINTS

■ When buying gotu kola supplements, look for those products that are standardized to contain 10% asiaticoside, an active ingredient in the herb. If you cannot find the standardized extract, you may substitute 400 to 500 mg of the crude herb for each 200 mg dose of the standardized extract.

FACTS & TIPS

■ Gotu kola is also known as *Centella asiatica*, talepetrako, Indian pennywort, Indian water navelwort, or hydrocotyle. A plant native to Europe, marsh pennywort (*Hydrocotyle vulgaris*), is a related species, but it has no known therapeutic properties.

■ Though the names sound similar, there's no relationship between gotu kola and the kola (or cola) nut, which is used in cola soft drinks. The kola nut is a stimulant containing caffeine; gotu kola is a very mild sedative and caffeine-free.

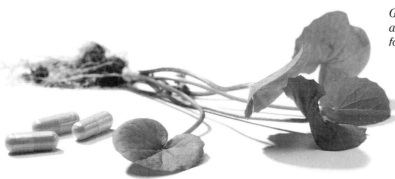

Gotu kola leaf is sold in a variety of supplement forms, including capsules.

GRAPE SEED EXTRACT

With antioxidant properties many times more powerful than those found in better-known nutrients (including vitamin C and vitamin E), grape seed extract is a heart-smart and cancer-smart botanical. It also has the power to improve vascular health, protect brain cells, and increase your overall well-being in myriad ways.

COMMON USES

- Treats blood vessel disorders.
- Protects against vision damage.
- Lessens the risk of heart disease and cancer.
- Reduces the rate of collagen breakdown in the skin.

FORMS

- Capsule
- Tablet
- Liquid

▼ WHAT IT IS

This extract made from the tiny seeds of red grapes is a flavonoid and one of Europe's leading natural treatments. Plant substances with potent antioxidant potential, flavonoids protect the cells from damage by unstable oxygen molecules called free radicals.

Grape seed extract contains procyanidolic oligomers (PCOs), also called proanthocyanidins. Once called pycnogenols (pik-NODGE-en-alls), PCOs are believed to play an important role in preventing heart disease and cancer.

"Pycnogenol" with a capital P is the trademark for a specific PCO derived from maritime pine bark; it can be used in place of grape seed extract, but it is more expensive, and many practitioners don't believe it's worth the extra cost.

▼ WHAT IT DOES

Grape seed extract exerts a powerful, positive influence on blood vessels. Not coincidentally, the active substances in this extract, PCOs, are key ingredients in one of the drugs most frequently prescribed for blood vessel (vascular) disorders in western Europe.

Because grape seed extract is both oil- and water-soluble, it can penetrate all types of cell membranes, delivering antioxidant protection throughout the body. Moreover, it is one of the few substances that can cross the blood-brain barrier, which means it has the potential to protect brain cells from free-radical damage.

MAJOR BENEFITS

With its powerful ability to enhance the health of blood vessels, grape seed extract may reduce the risk of heart attack and stroke and also strengthen fragile or weak capillaries and increase blood flow, particularly to the extremities. For this reason, many experts find it a beneficial supplement for almost any type of vascular insufficiency, as well as for conditions that are associated with poor vascular function, including diabetes, varicose veins, some cases of impotence, numbness and tingling in the arms and legs, and even painful leg cramps.

Because it can have an impact on even the tiniest blood vessels, grape seed

 ALERT

SIDE EFFECTS
- No side effects from taking grape seed extract have been reported, and no toxic reactions have been noted.

CAUTION
- **Reminder:** If you have a medical condition, talk to your doctor before taking supplements.

extract also benefits circulation in the eye. It is frequently recommended as a supplement to combat macular degeneration and cataracts, two of the most common causes of blindness in older people. And if you use computers on a regular basis, grape seed extract may also be for you. At least one study showed that 300 mg daily for just 60 days reduced eyestrain associated with computer monitor work and improved contrast vision.

Many experts now endorse grape seed extract for its cancer-fighting properties. Working as antioxidants, PCOs correct damage to the genetic material of cells that could possibly cause tumors to form.

ADDITIONAL BENEFITS

Helping to preserve and reinforce the collagen in the skin, grape seed extract is often used in the treatment of connective tissue disorders, such as rheumatoid arthritis. In Europe, it is often included in cosmetic creams to improve skin elasticity.

For allergy sufferers, grape seed extract offers relief; it inhibits the release of symptom-causing compounds such as histamine, which, in turn, helps control a variety of allergic reactions, from hives to hay fever. Grape seed also blocks the release of prostaglandins, chemicals involved in allergic reactions and in pain and inflammation, particularly that of endometriosis, a menstrual disorder.

▼ HOW TO TAKE IT

DOSAGE

Choose supplements that are standardized to contain 92% to 95% proanthocyanidins, or PCOs.

For antioxidant protection: Take 100 mg daily.
For therapeutic benefits: Doses are usually 200 mg daily.

GUIDELINES FOR USE

• After 24 hours, only about 28% of grape seed extract's active components remain in the body. So it's important to take supplements at the same time every day, particularly when they are used to combat disease.

• Grape seed extract is best used with other antioxidants such as vitamins C and E; money-saving combination products are available.

FACTS & TIPS

■ Grape seed oil (not to be confused with grape seed extract) may offer health benefits too. A preliminary study at the University Health Science Center in Syracuse, New York, found that adding about 2 tablespoons of grape seed oil to the daily diet increased HDL ("good") cholesterol by 14% and reduced triglycerides by 15% in just four weeks. Try using it in place of other oils in salads or cooking.

LATEST FINDINGS

■ A preliminary study from the University of Arizona at Tucson suggests that pine bark extract, which contains the same active ingredients as grape seed extract, may be as effective an anticoagulant as aspirin, and so may help lower the risk of heart attack and stroke. Researchers asked 38 smokers—who are more likely to develop the type of blood clots that cause heart attacks—to take either pine bark extract or aspirin. Blood tests revealed that both remedies were equally effective, but pine bark did not have aspirin's side effects—such as stomach irritation and increased risk for internal bleeding.

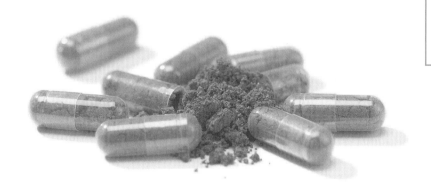

GREEN TEA *(Camellia sinensis)*

According to legend, around 2700 B.C. a Chinese emperor sat under a tea shrub, and a few leaves fell into his cup of hot water. Presto! Green tea was born. Now, modern research has found that this type of tea—a staple of the Asian diet—contains one of the most promising anticancer compounds ever discovered.

COMMON USES
- May help prevent cancer.
- Protects against heart disease.
- Inhibits tooth decay.
- Promotes longevity.

FORMS
- Capsule
- Tablet
- Liquid
- Powder
- Tea

▼ WHAT IT IS

The traditional process that yields green tea is simple: The leaves from the tea plant are first steamed, then rolled and dried. The steaming kills enzymes that would otherwise ferment the leaves.

With other types of tea, the leaves are allowed to ferment either partially (for oolong tea) or fully (for black tea). The lack of fermentation, however, gives green tea its unique flavor and, more important, preserves virtually all of the naturally present polyphenols (strong antioxidants that can protect against cell damage).

Other substances in green tea that also appear to have medicinal properties are fluoride, catechins, and tannins.

▼ WHAT IT DOES

Green tea possesses compounds that may provide powerful protection against several cancers and, possibly, against heart disease. Studies indicate that it also fights infection and promotes longevity.

PREVENTION
The rate of certain types of cancer is lower among people who drink green tea. In one large-scale study, researchers found that Chinese men and women who drank green tea as seldom as once a week for six months had lower rates of rectal, pancreatic, and possibly colon cancer than those who rarely or never drank it. In women, the risk of rectal and pancreatic cancer was nearly cut in half. Preliminary research suggests that green tea may also fight breast, stomach, and skin cancer.

Studies investigating how green tea might guard against cancer have pointed to the potency of its main antioxidant, a polyphenol dubbed EGCG (for epigallocatechin-gallate). Some scientists believe EGCG may be one of the most effective anticancer compounds ever discovered, protecting cells from damage and strengthening the body's own production of antioxidant enzymes.

According to a study from Ohio's Case Western Reserve University, EGCG seems to signal cancer cells to stop

ALERT

SIDE EFFECTS
• Green tea is very safe, both as a supplement and as a beverage. People who are sensitive to caffeine, however, may not want to drink too much green tea, because each cup contains about 40 mg of caffeine.

• Because of its caffeine content, pregnant women and those who are breast-feeding should limit their green tea consumption to two cups a day.

CAUTION
• **Reminder:** If you have a medical condition, talk to your doctor before taking supplements.

reproducing by stimulating a natural process of programmed cell death called apoptosis. Remarkably, EGCG does not harm healthy cells. In addition, research at the Medical College of Ohio indicates that EGCG inhibits the production of urokinase, an enzyme that cancer cells need in order to grow. In animals, blocking urokinase shrinks tumors and sometimes causes cancer to go into complete remission.

ADDITIONAL BENEFITS

The antioxidant effect of green tea's polyphenols may also help protect the heart. In test-tube studies, these compounds appeared to suppress the blood-vessel damage due to LDL cholesterol, thought to be an initial step in the buildup of plaque in the arteries. A Japanese study of 1,371 men linked daily green tea consumption to the prevention of heart disease.

In addition, green tea contains fluoride, which may help to protect against tooth decay, and provides an overall antibacterial effect.

▼ HOW TO TAKE IT

DOSAGE

You can get the benefits of green tea by taking either green tea capsules or tablets or by drinking several cups of the brew each day. Your aim should be to get 240 to 320 mg of polyphenols.

When using supplements, buy those standardized to contain at least 50% polyphenols. At this concentration, two 250 mg supplements would provide 250 mg of polyphenols. Studies show that four cups of freshly brewed green tea also supply the recommended amount of polyphenols.

Green tea supplements have very little caffeine. The recommended dose of green tea supplements provides the same amount of polyphenols as four cups of green tea, but generally contains only 5 to 6 mg of caffeine.

GUIDELINES FOR USE

• Take green tea supplements at meals with a full glass of water.

• Drink freshly brewed green tea on its own or with meals. To make the tea, use 1 teaspoon of green tea leaves per cup of very hot (but not boiling) water. Let the brew steep for three to five minutes; then strain and drink it.

Green tea can be taken in supplement form or enjoyed as a soothing beverage.

FACTS & TIPS

■ Green tea leaves contain hefty amounts of vitamin K, but a cup of brewed tea or green tea supplements have virtually none. This means that people taking anti-coagulant drugs for heart disease (who may have been told to avoid large servings of foods rich in vitamin K because of the vitamin's influence on blood clotting) can enjoy green tea with no fear of side effects.

■ Drinking boiling hot green tea can damage your throat and esophagus and may over time increase your cancer risk. Try the traditional Asian method: Heat cold water until just before it boils (or boil it and let it cool for a few minutes), then pour the hot (but not boiling) water over the tea leaves. This method also helps accent the delicate flavor of green tea.

■ Imported from China, gunpowder tea is simply green tea presented in tiny pellets resembling gunpowder. When placed in hot water, the leaves slowly unfold.

LATEST FINDINGS

■ According to researchers at the University of Kansas, green tea's main antioxidant (EGCG) is 100 times more powerful than vitamin C and 25 times more potent than vitamin E in protecting DNA from the kind of damage thought to increase cancer risk.

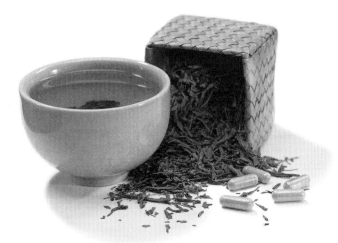

GUGULIPID *(Commiphora mukul)*

Since antiquity, practitioners of Ayurvedic medicine in India have used the gum resin of the mukul myrrh tree to treat obesity and arthritis. Now a modern purified extract called gugulipid has been found to be as effective as some prescription drugs for lowering cholesterol and trigliceride levels in the blood.

COMMON USES

- Helps lower high blood cholesterol and high blood triglycerides.
- Reduces heart disease risk.
- Treats arthritis inflammation.
- May aid weight loss.

FORMS

- Capsule
- Tablet
- Powder

▼ WHAT IT IS

Gugulipid comes from the gummy resin of the small thorny mukul myrrh tree native to India. The tree's resin is closely related to the richly perfumed Biblical myrrh, traditionally used for purification purposes.

Called gum guggul ("guggulu"), the resin itself has been part of Ayurveda, the traditional medicine of India, for thousands of years. Guggulu, however, has toxic compounds. Fortunately, modern Indian pharmacologists have devised a way to extract the active components in the resins and leave the toxic substances behind. The result is the standardized extract called gugulipid.

▼ WHAT IT DOES

The active ingredients in gugulipid, known as guggulsterones, appear to affect the way the body metabolizes fat and cholesterol. These compounds also have anti-inflammatory and anti-oxidant properties.

PREVENTION

If you have high blood cholesterol levels, you are at increased risk for developing coronary heart disease. Studies suggest that gugulipid can lower these levels; it is the guggulsterones, in particular, that seem to stimulate the liver to break down the most harmful form of cholesterol, LDL.

In addition, gugulipid sometimes elevates the levels of protective HDL cholesterol. A study of 205 people in India found that gugulipid, in combination with a low-fat diet, reduced total cholesterol by an average of 24% in more than three-quarters of the participants.

In another study comparing the efficacy of gugulipid with that of clofibrate, a prescription cholesterol-lowering medication, total cholesterol dropped by 11% in the gugulipid group and by 10% in the clofibrate group. In addition, nearly two-thirds of those taking gugulipid experienced increases in HDL cholesterol levels on average; however, no change in HDL was seen in those using clofibrate.

 ALERT

SIDE EFFECTS
- Rarely, taking gugulipid may cause minor gastrointestinal problems, such as mild nausea, gas, or hiccups. In a few cases, headaches have also been reported.

CAUTION
- Never use the crude gum guggul, or guggulu, which can cause rashes, diarrhea, stomach pain, and loss of appetite. Opt for the standardized gugulipid products instead.

- Be sure to consult your doctor before trying gugulipid if you suffer from liver disease, inflammatory bowel disease, or diarrhea.

- Pregnant women should not use gugulipid.

- **Reminder:** If you have a medical condition, talk to your doctor before taking supplements.

In animal studies, gugulipid has been shown to prevent the formation of artery-blocking plaque, and even to help reverse existing plaque. In addition, it inhibits blood platelets from sticking together, and thus may protect against blood clots, which often trigger heart attacks.

ADDITIONAL BENEFITS

Studies lend support to two of the traditional uses for guggul: treating arthritis and obesity.

Results from animal studies indicate that the anti-inflammatory action of guggulsterones may be as powerful as that of over-the-counter pain medications, such as ibuprofen, making this herb useful in treating arthritis. Its anti-inflammatory action also suggests that gugulipid may be effective for acne; in fact, one study showed it had a beneficial effect on this condition.

There is some evidence that gugulipid stimulates the production of thyroid hormones, increasing the rate at which the body burns calories. In one small study, Indian researchers reported that in overweight patients, gugulipid supplements sparked significant weight loss. Much of the weight loss came from a reduction in fat around the abdomen, which is associated with an increased risk of heart disease and diabetes. Any effective long-term weight control program, of course, must begin with a low-fat, high-fiber diet and a regular exercise program.

▼ HOW TO TAKE IT

DOSAGE

To lower cholesterol: Take a supplement that supplies 25 mg of guggulsterones per dose, three times a day.

GUIDELINES FOR USE

• You can take gugulipid with or without meals.

• Don't stop seeing your doctor for a cholesterol problem, and on your own never substitute a gugulipid product for a cholesterol-lowering medication without getting your doctor's approval first.

LATEST FINDINGS

■ Gugulipid may act as an antioxidant with heart-protective qualities. Because LDL cholesterol is most harmful when it's been damaged by unstable oxygen molecules called free radicals, protecting LDL from oxidation may help prevent heart disease. In a study of 61 patients with high cholesterol levels, 31 were given gugulipid (100 mg of guggulsterones a day) and 30 took a placebo. After 24 weeks, those taking gugulipid had a 13% drop in LDL cholesterol and a 12% drop in triglycerides, whereas the placebo group experienced no change. Furthermore, researchers found that the susceptibility of LDL cholesterol to free-radical damage declined by a third in the gugulipid group, but there was no change in the placebo group.

DID YOU KNOW?

As early as 600 B.C., Ayurvedic physicians in India described a disease marked by the overeating of fatty foods, lack of exercise, an impaired metabolism, and the "coating and obstruction of channels." They called it "medoroga" (today it's known as atherosclerosis); to treat it they used guggul, a precursor to gugulipid.

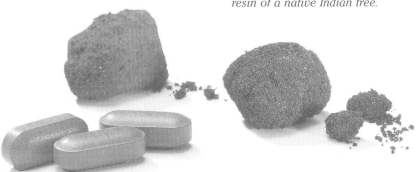

Gugulipid supplements are derived from the dark gummy resin of a native Indian tree.

HAWTHORN *(Crataegus oxyacantha)*

If your doctor confirms that you have any form of heart disease, you'll want to know all about hawthorn. Historically used as a diuretic and as a treatment for kidney and bladder stones, this herb today is widely prescribed in Europe as a natural heart remedy for conditions ranging from mild hypertension to angina.

COMMON USES

- Relieves chest pain of angina.
- Lowers high blood pressure.
- Helps the heart pump more efficiently in people with congestive heart failure.
- Corrects irregular heartbeat (cardiac arrhythmia).

FORMS

- Tablet
- Capsule
- Liquid
- Powder
- Dried herb/Tea

▼ WHAT IT IS

For centuries, hawthorn, a shrub that grows to 30 feet, has been trimmed to hedge height and planted along the edges of fields or property lines. As a divider, it looks attractive and discourages trespassers: It produces pretty white flowers and vibrant red berries, but it also sports large thorns, and the flowers on some varieties smell like rotting meat.

What's more, the plant has long been associated with bad luck and death, because the crown of thorns that Christ wore at the Crucifixion is widely believed to have been woven from hawthorn twigs.

Given this reputation, it's surprising that anyone got close enough to discover hawthorn's cardioprotective benefits. But obviously a number of people in different eras and locations—from the ancient Greeks to the Native Americans—did consider the herb a potent tonic for the heart.

The modern use of hawthorn originated with a nineteenth-century Irish physician who treated heart disease quite successfully. Because he closely guarded his heart formula, not until after his death in the 1890s was his secret remedy revealed to be tincture of hawthorn berry.

▼ WHAT IT DOES

Hawthorn is an herb that directly benefits the workings of the heart. It can help dilate blood vessels, increase the heart's energy supply, and improve its pumping ability. These powerful cardiac effects can probably be traced to hawthorn's abundant supply of plant compounds called flavonoids—and especially procyanidolic oligomers (PCOs), which are potent antioxidants.

MAJOR BENEFITS

Hawthorn seems to be an all-purpose heart drug. It widens arteries by interfering with an enzyme called ACE (angiotensin-converting enzyme), which constricts blood vessels. This action improves blood flow through

ALERT

SIDE EFFECTS

- Though there have been reports of nausea, sweating, fatigue, and skin rash, these side effects are uncommon. Stop taking the herb and consult your doctor if any of these reactions occur.

- In people who don't have heart disease, large doses of hawthorn can cause very low blood pressure, which can lead to dizziness and fainting.

CAUTION

- Hawthorn appears to be safe to use with most drugs prescribed for heart disease. Talk with your doctor before trying hawthorn, and never stop taking a drug that's been prescribed for you (or reduce the dose) without your doctor's consent.

- Chest pain (angina) is a very serious symptom of heart trouble; don't expect hawthorn to stop an acute angina attack. See your doctor.

- **Reminder:** If you have a medical condition, talk to your doctor before taking supplements.

the arteries, making the herb a good remedy for people with angina.

In addition, because chronically constricted arteries can lead to high blood pressure (they force the heart to work harder to pump blood through inflexible blood vessels), hawthorn may reduce blood pressure in individuals with mild hypertension.

Hawthorn also seems to block enzymes that weaken the heart muscle, thereby strengthening its pumping power. This property is especially useful for individuals with mild congestive heart failure who don't require strong heart medications, such as digitalis. Moreover, the antioxidant properties of hawthorn may help protect against damage associated with the buildup of plaque in the coronary arteries.

ADDITIONAL BENEFITS

Hawthorn has a long history as a treatment for other conditions as well. It seems to exert a calming effect and functions as a sleeping aid in some who suffer from insomnia. Several researchers have also noted that hawthorn preserves collagen—the protein that composes connective tissue—which is damaged in such diseases as arthritis.

▼ HOW TO TAKE IT

DOSAGE

The recommended dose of hawthorn extract ranges from 300 to 450 mg a day in pill form, and from 1 teaspoon to 1 tablespoon (5 to 15 ml) of the liquid extract, depending on the type of heart condition.

People at risk for heart disease may wish to take a 100 to 150 mg supplement or 1 teaspoon of the liquid extract daily as a heart disease preventive.

GUIDELINES FOR USE

• If you're on large doses, hawthorn works best when the daily amount is divided and taken at three different times during the day.

• Hawthorn may take a couple of months to build up in your system before it produces noticeable results.

SHOPPING HINTS

■ When buying hawthorn, look for standardized extracts that contain at least 1.8% vitexin, sometimes called vitexin-2-rhamnoside. This is the main heart-protective substance in the herb.

LATEST FINDINGS

■ In an eight-week German study of 136 people with mild to moderate congestive heart failure, those who took hawthorn extract reported less shortness of breath, less ankle swelling, and better exercise performance than those given a placebo. Physical exams and laboratory tests confirmed that the condition of the hawthorn group improved while the condition of the placebo group worsened.

DID YOU KNOW?

Hawthorn varieties grow in Europe, eastern Asia, northern Africa, and the United States. It is also known as whitethorn and mayflower—in fact, the Pilgrim ship the *Mayflower* was named after the hawthorn blossom.

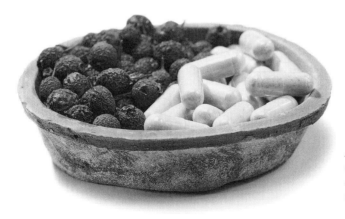

Hawthorn supplements may contain the plant's leaves and flowers, its red berries, or a combination of all three.

IODINE

Many people associate iodine with the orange-brown topical antiseptic their mothers swabbed on their childhood scrapes and bruises. But the real value of this potent trace mineral is its role in the health of the thyroid gland, where it is involved in numerous biological functions that we couldn't live without.

COMMON USES
■ Corrects an iodine deficiency.
■ Ensures proper functioning of the thyroid gland.
■ May help treat fibrocystic breasts.

FORMS
■ Tablet
■ Capsule
■ Liquid

▼ WHAT IT IS

Although the body needs just tiny amounts of iodine, this mineral is so crucial to an individual's overall health that in the 1920s government officials decided it should be added to a foodstuff common to nearly everyone—namely, table salt. The introduction of iodized salt to the American diet virtually eliminated one severe form of mental retardation called cretinism.

Despite the recognized importance of this vital mineral, however, about 1.6 billion people in the world, mostly in underdeveloped countries, still suffer from iodine deficiency.

▼ WHAT IT DOES

Unique among minerals, iodine has only one known function in the body: It is essential to the thyroid gland for manufacturing thyroxine, a hormone that regulates metabolism in all the body's cells.

PREVENTION
By getting enough iodine, pregnant women can prevent certain types of mental retardation in the fetus.

ADDITIONAL BENEFITS
Unlike many other minerals, iodine does not seem to help in the treatment of specific diseases; however, it does play a fundamental role in assuring the health of the thyroid, the butterfly-shaped gland that surrounds the windpipe (trachea).

When your iodine intake is adequate, your body contains about an ounce of it, and 75% of that amount is stored in the thyroid. This organ controls the body's overall metabolism, which determines how quickly and efficiently calories are burned. It also regulates growth and development in children, reproduction, nerve and muscle function, the breakdown of proteins and fats, the growth of nails and hair, and the use of oxygen by every cell in the body.

There is some evidence that iodine derived from an organic source may be effective in reducing the pain of fibrocystic breasts, but patients should discuss this type of supplementation with their doctor first.

▼ HOW MUCH YOU NEED

The RDA for iodine is 150 mcg daily for adult men and women. Most

ALERT

CAUTION
• Because iodine deficiency is rare in developed countries, take iodine supplements only if prescribed by your physician.

• **Reminder:** If you have a medical or psychiatric condition, talk to your doctor before taking supplements.

people meet or exceed this amount by using iodized salt (1 teaspoon of iodized salt contains more than 300 mcg of iodine).

IF YOU GET TOO LITTLE
Thanks to the widespread use of iodized salt, not a single case of iodine deficiency has been reported in the United States since the 1970s.

Among the first signs of iodine deficiency, now rarely seen, is an enlarged thyroid gland, known as a goiter. Lack of iodine can cause the gland to expand in an attempt to increase its surface area and trap as much of the iodine in the bloodstream as possible.

If your iodine intake is low, your thyroid hormone level may well be low too. This condition can lead to fatigue, dry skin, a rise in blood fats, a hoarse voice, delayed reflexes, and reduced mental clarity. See your doctor if you have these symptoms.

IF YOU GET TOO MUCH
There is very little risk of iodine overdose, even at levels 10 to 20 times the RDA. However, if you ingest 30 times the RDA, you are likely to experience a metallic taste, mouth sores, swollen salivary glands, diarrhea, vomiting, headache, a rash, and difficulty in breathing. Ironically, a goiter can also develop if you consistently take extremely large amounts of iodine.

▼ HOW TO TAKE IT

DOSAGE
You probably get all the iodine you need from iodized salt or from regular servings of seafood. Iodine is also a standard ingredient in many multivitamin and mineral supplements.

Even if you are on a strict, very low salt diet for high blood pressure, you probably don't require extra iodine, though you can safely take 150 mcg a day.

People taking a thyroid hormone should always discuss their condition with a doctor before taking individual iodine supplements.

GUIDELINES FOR USE
• When prescribed, iodine supplements can be taken at any time of the day, with or without food.

▼ OTHER SOURCES

Although the most abundant source of iodine is iodized table salt, the mineral can also be found in saltwater fish and in sea vegetation, such as kelp. Soil in coastal areas also tends to be iodine-rich, as are the dairy products produced by cows grazing there. The same is true for fruits and vegetables grown in soil high in iodine.

Commercial baked goods—such as breads and cakes—are other good sources of iodine. Though iodized salt is not used in commercial baking, these products are often made with dough conditioners that contain iodine.

FACTS & TIPS
■ Even though health-food stores frequently promote sea salt as a healthier alternative to table salt, sea salt is not iodized, and so is not a good source of iodine.

■ If you're thinking that the pretzels or potato chips you nosh on are probably providing all the iodine you need, guess again. Iodized salt isn't used to flavor popular salty snacks.

LATEST FINDINGS
■ An analysis of 10 different studies performed in countries where iodine deficiency is common found evidence that an iodine deficiency can affect motor skills, decreasing reaction time, manual dexterity, coordination, and muscle strength. The analysis, headed by UNICEF researchers, also revealed that the IQ of people who were iodine deficient was some 13 points below that of those who had an adequate iodine intake.

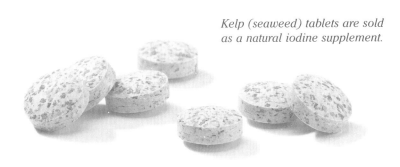

Kelp (seaweed) tablets are sold as a natural iodine supplement.

IRON

A surprising number of Americans get too little iron—and few realize that a lack of this vital mineral can make them weak, unable to concentrate, and more susceptible to infection. Too much iron, however, can be dangerous. A blood test can show whether you would benefit from an iron supplement.

COMMON USES

■ Treats iron-deficiency anemia.

■ Often needed during pregnancy; by women with heavy menstrual periods; or in other situations determined by your doctor.

FORMS

■ Tablet

■ Capsule

■ Softgel

■ Liquid

▼ WHAT IT IS

Needed throughout the body, iron is an essential part of hemoglobin, the oxygen-carrying component of red blood cells. The mineral is also found in myoglobin, which supplies oxygen to the muscles of the body, and is part of many important enzymes and immune-system compounds.

The body, which gets most of the iron it requires from foods, carefully monitors its iron status, absorbing more of the mineral when demand is high (during periods of rapid growth, such as pregnancy or childhood) and less when stores of it are adequate.

Because the body loses iron when bleeding, many menstruating women have low iron levels. Dieters, vegetarians, and endurance athletes may experience iron shortfalls as well.

▼ WHAT IT DOES

By helping the blood and muscles deliver oxygen, iron supplies energy to every cell in the body. Yet iron deficiency is surprisingly common in the United States. According to federal statistics, 9% of adolescent girls and 11% of women under age 50 are deficient in this mineral.

Though it is very difficult to develop an iron deficiency from poor nutrition (iron is found in many foods), women with heavy menstrual periods and people with certain medical conditions may need supplements to prevent or correct the severe condition known as iron-deficiency anemia.

MAJOR BENEFITS
Keeping your body well supplied with iron provides energy, helps your immune system function at its best, and gives your mind an edge. Studies show that even mild iron deficiency—well short of the levels commonly associated with anemia—can cause adults to have a short attention span and teens to do poorly in school.

▼ HOW MUCH YOU NEED

The RDA for iron in men of all ages and women over age 50 is 8 mg a day. For younger women, it's 18 mg daily (in pregnancy, 27 mg a day). To combat anemia, additional iron—either

▲ ALERT ▲
CAUTION
• Never take an iron supplement unless you are following your doctor's recommendation. More than one million Americans have an inherited disease called hemochromatosis, whish causes them to absorb too much iron—and most don't even know it. (Early symptoms include fatigue and aching joints.)

• Taking iron on your own could mask a cause of anemia, such as a bleeding ulcer, and prevent a doctor from making an early, lifesaving diagnosis.

• **Reminder:** If you have a medical condition, talk to your doctor before taking supplements.

through diet or supplements—is typically needed for a period of weeks or months.

IF YOU GET TOO LITTLE

If you get too little iron in your diet or lose too much through heavy menstrual periods, stomach bleeding (commonly caused by arthritis drugs), or cancer, your body draws on its iron reserve. Initially, there are no symptoms, but as your iron supply dwindles, so does your body's ability to produce healthy red blood cells. The result is iron-deficiency anemia, marked by weakness, fatigue, paleness, breathlessness, palpitations, and increased susceptibility to infection.

IF YOU GET TOO MUCH

Some studies link too much iron to an increased risk of chronic diseases, including heart disease and colon cancer. Excess iron can be particularly dangerous for adults with a genetic tendency to overabsorb it (hemochromatosis), and for children, who are especially susceptible to iron overdose.

▼ HOW TO TAKE IT

DOSAGE

Iron supplements should be taken only under your doctor's supervision; self-treatment can be dangerous. Anemia requires a careful diagnosis and treatment to correct the underlying cause.

When a doctor recommends it, iron is typically taken in a form called ferrous salts—usually ferrous sulfate, ferrous fumarate, or ferrous gluconate. A typical prescribed dose provides about 30 mg of iron one to three times daily.

Most men and postmenopausal women do not need iron supplements and should make sure iron is not included in their daily multivitamin.

GUIDELINES FOR USE

• Iron is best absorbed when taken on an empty stomach. If iron upsets your stomach, have it with meals, preferably with a small amount of meat and a food or drink rich in vitamin C, such as broccoli or orange juice, to help boost the amount of iron your body absorbs.

• Never take iron for more than six months without having your blood iron levels rechecked by your doctor.

▼ OTHER SOURCES

Iron-rich foods include liver, beef, and lamb. Clams, oysters, and mussels also contain iron.

Vegetarians can get plenty of iron from beans and peas, leafy greens, dried fruits (apricots, raisins), seeds (pumpkin, squash, sunflower), and fortified breakfast cereals. Brewer's yeast, kelp, blackstrap molasses, and wheat bran are also exceptionally good sources.

Cooking tomatoes or other acidic foods in a cast-iron pot adds iron to meals as well; a healthful amount leaches out of the cookware into the food.

SHOPPING HINTS

■ One of the most common forms of iron supplement (ferrous sulfate) is inexpensive, but it can cause constipation and stomach upset. Other forms, such as ferrous fumarate or ferrous gluconate, may be easier to tolerate. Iron-rich herbal tonics, which are sold in health-food stores, may be even gentler.

■ Check the labels on any multivitamin and mineral supplements you take to see if you're getting extra iron. If you're not at risk for anemia, you probably don't need it—and it could be hazardous.

FACTS & TIPS

■ Keep all supplements containing iron out of reach of children. Just five high-potency iron pills can kill a small child.

■ Iron supplements can interfere with the effects of antibiotics and other medications. Be sure to tell your doctor about any supplements you are taking in addition to your regular medications.

■ Women who are even slightly deficient in iron feel cold sooner than women with adequate blood levels of iron. For them, taking iron supplements is truly heart-warming.

DID YOU KNOW?

Younger women would have to eat about 15 snack-size boxes of raisins daily to get the 15 mg of iron recommended for them.

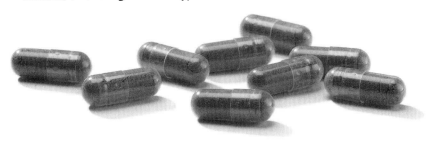

KAVA *(Piper methysticum)*

When English explorer Captain James Cook sailed the South Pacific in the 1700s, the kava-laced drink his crew sampled on tropical islands along the way may have eased the stress of the long journey. The herb has long been appreciated for its calming effects, and today it continues to attract new enthusiasts.

COMMON USES
- Combats anxiety.
- Eases panic attacks.
- Helps induce sleep.
- Relieves pain.

FORMS
- Capsule
- Tablet
- Softgel
- Liquid
- Dried herb/Tea

▼ WHAT IT IS

A member of the pepper family, kava (also known as kava-kava) is a shrub that thrives on many South Pacific islands. The name "kava" refers not only to the herb but also to a traditional beverage made by crushing the plant's root into a pulp, adding water or coconut milk, and straining it into coconut shells.

For thousands of years, kava has played a major role in social events and religious rituals among Pacific islanders. In fact, island ceremonies—whether those welcoming royalty or simply hosting a neighborhood get-together—wouldn't be complete without kava, which serves a purpose similar to that of alcohol in other societies, namely, inducing a sense of well-being and fostering social discourse.

The kava plant, with its heart-shaped leaves, bears sterile flowers and can be propagated only by dividing the roots, which are thick and gnarled. These can weigh up to 22 pounds. Today in many parts of the South Pacific, kava is widely cultivated for the medicinal properties of its roots and is exported to herb shops throughout the world.

▼ WHAT IT DOES

Kava root contains a number of compounds (the most prominent are known as kavalactones), which have a wide range of therapeutic effects. In many European countries, doctors currently prescribe kava for the treatment of anxiety, stress, restlessness, and insomnia. Scientists aren't sure how it works but believe that kava targets the limbic system, a primitive part of the brain that (among other things) regulates emotions.

MAJOR BENEFITS
Kava is known primarily for its anxiety-relieving benefits. It can be useful for

ALERT

SIDE EFFECTS
- Stomach upset is the most common side effect. Occasionally, very high doses for extended periods (at least three months) can cause the skin to turn yellow (first the face, then the body) and to become dry and scaly.

- Very high doses may also cause loss of appetite, labored breathing, blurred vision, bloodshot eyes, walking difficulties, and intoxication. If any of these reactions occur, stop taking kava.

CAUTION
- Unless your doctor recommends it, avoid this herb if you are regularly taking other drugs that affect the central nervous system, such as antidepressants, sedatives, or tranquilizers.

- Don't take more than the recommended dose. Higher doses can cause disorientation or intoxication, and even recommended doses taken for more than three months can increase the risk of adverse reactions.

- Pregnant or breast-feeding women should not use kava.

- Don't take kava if you have Parkinson's disease. It may increase symptoms.

- Avoid alcohol while taking kava.

- **Reminder:** If you have a medical or psychiatric condition, talk to your doctor before taking supplements.

reducing general stress and nervousness, as well as for warding off the intense bouts of anxiety known as panic attacks. Kava can also have a calming, sedative effect on individuals who are trying to stop smoking or wean themselves off alcohol. Its relaxing properties may help insomniacs fall asleep. And those with mild to moderate depression, who often suffer from anxiety, may likewise benefit from the herb's properties.

Unlike conventional tranquilizers, kava doesn't appear to dull the mind. Some studies even show that it improves mental reaction time. Surprisingly, people taking kava rarely seem to develop a tolerance to the herb. Also, kava generally doesn't seem to be addictive.

ADDITIONAL BENEFITS
Kava has pain-relieving qualities that may be of value in treating muscle aches as well as chronic pain affecting any part of the body. It also appears to have muscle-relaxing properties, and so may be beneficial for easing painful muscle spasms.

In some people with epilepsy, kava seems to prevent seizures as effectively as some prescription anticonvulsants; its effects may be related to its power to relieve stress and anxiety, which can trigger epileptic attacks. Furthermore, preliminary studies suggest the herb may help stroke patients recover by minimizing the amount of permanent brain damage that can occur.

▼ HOW TO TAKE IT

DOSAGE
The recommended dose is 250 mg of a standardized extract two or three times a day. Consult your doctor if you have been taking kava for more than three months because prolonged use increases the chance of side effects.

GUIDELINES FOR USE
• Do not exceed the recommended dose. Higher dosages can lead to intoxication or disorientation. One man in Utah, for instance, was convicted of driving under the influence after spending the evening consuming 16 cups of kava tea, which caused him to stagger, slur his speech, and drive as if drunk on alcohol.

• Look for extracts standardized to contain at least 30% of the herb's active ingredients, which are called kavalactones. Or look for products containing kavapyrones—another name for the active ingredient—which varies with preparation. Most human studies used 70 to 240 mg kavapyrones daily.

• Kava is sometimes combined with herbal supplements that affect the brain, such as the antidepressant St. John's wort.

• Kava usually acts within minutes, though for some people with severe anxiety, the full benefits may not be apparent until up to eight weeks after first consuming the herb.

SHOPPING HINTS
■ Buy kava that's been extracted from the root of the plant—and not a product that has only purified kavalactones. The root extracts appear to contain a blend of beneficial substances, in addition to kavalactones.

LATEST FINDINGS
■ In a major study conducted at several European medical centers, 101 patients with anxiety took either 100 mg of kava extract three times a day or a placebo. After 24 weeks, 76% of those in the kava group said that they were "much" or "very much" improved, compared to 51% of those getting a placebo. The study found it took eight weeks before there was any significant benefit from kava (earlier studies had indicated some benefit after four weeks or less) perhaps because the patients in this study were suffering from severe and long-term anxiety. The only side effect that researchers noted was an occasional upset stomach.

DID YOU KNOW?
During South Pacific welcoming ceremonies, Lyndon and Lady Bird Johnson, Hillary Rodham Clinton, Queen Elizabeth, and Pope John Paul II all drank kava.

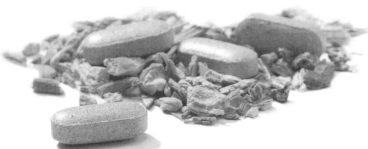

The dried root of the tropical kava plant can be made into stress-relieving pills or a soothing tea.

LECITHIN and CHOLINE

These closely related nutrients are members of the vitamin B family, and though you may never have heard of them, they are actually essential for every cell in your body. Because they are particularly important for the liver and nerves, it's not surprising that so many nutritionists urge Americans to get more of them.

COMMON USES

- Help in preventing gallstones.
- Strengthen the liver, making them useful in the treatment of hepatitis and cirrhosis.
- Aid the liver in ridding the body of toxins in patients undergoing chemotherapy for cancer.
- Diminish heartburn symptoms.
- May boost memory and enhance brain function.

FORMS

- Capsule
- Tablet
- Softgel
- Powder/Grains
- Liquid

▼ WHAT IT IS

Lecithin (pronounced LESS-a-thin) is a fatty substance found in many animal- and plant-based foods, including liver, eggs, soybeans, peanuts, and wheat germ. It is often added to processed foods—including ice cream, chocolate, margarine, and salad dressings—to help blend, or emulsify, the fats with water. In addition, the body manufactures its own supply as well.

Lecithin is considered an excellent source of the B vitamin choline, primarily in the form called phosphatidylcholine. Once in the body, phosphatidylcholine breaks down into choline, so that when you take lecithin, or absorb lecithin from foods, your body gets choline.

Only 10% to 20% of the lecithin found in plants and other natural sources consists of phosphatidylcholine. You can buy lecithin supplements that contain higher concentrations of phosphatidylcholine, but they can be very expensive. For most situations, just taking plain lecithin, rather than the more costly phosphatidylcholine, works fine.

Though dietary lecithin is a primary source of choline, choline is also found in liver, soybeans, egg yolks, grape juice, peanuts, cabbage, cauliflower, and other foods. You can also buy choline supplements, and choline is often included as an ingredient in B-complex vitamins or other combination formulas.

▼ WHAT IT DOES

Lecithin and choline are needed for a range of body functions. They help build cell membranes and facilitate the movement of fats and nutrients in and out of cells. They aid in reproduction and in fetal and infant development; they're essential to liver and gallbladder health; and they may help the heart. Choline is also a key component of the brain chemical acetylcholine, which plays a major role in memory and muscle control.

As a result of these far-flung effects, lecithin and choline have been touted for almost everything—from curing cancer and AIDS to lowering cholesterol. And even though the evidence

ALERT

SIDE EFFECTS
- In high doses, lecithin and choline may cause sweating, nausea, vomiting, bloating, and diarrhea. Taking very high dosages of choline (10 grams a day) may produce a fishy body odor or a heart rhythm disorder.

CAUTION
- Because individual lecithin, choline, or phosphatidylcholine supplements can increase levels of acetylcholine, they should not be used by people who are suffering from bipolar disorder. High levels of acetylcholine can worsen the "depressive" stage of the condition.

- **Reminder:** If you have a medical or psychiatric condition, talk to your doctor before taking supplements.

for some of these claims is weak, these nutrients should not be dismissed out of hand.

MAJOR BENEFITS
Lecithin and choline may be especially helpful in the treatment of gallbladder and liver diseases. Lecithin is a key component of bile, the fat-digesting substance, and low levels of this nutrient are known to precipitate gallstones. Taking supplements with lecithin or its purified extract, phosphatidylcholine, may treat or prevent this disorder.

Lecithin may also be beneficial for the liver: The results of a 10-year study on baboons showed that it prevented severe liver scarring and cirrhosis caused by alcohol abuse; other studies have indicated that it helps liver problems associated with hepatitis.

Choline is often included in liver complex formulas along with other liver-strengthening supplements, such as the B vitamin inositol, the amino acid methionine, and the herbs milk thistle and dandelion. These preparations, often called lipotropic combinations or factors, can protect against the buildup of fats within the liver, improve the flow of fats and cholesterol through the liver and gallbladder, and help the liver rid the body of dangerous toxins.

Lecithin and choline may be especially helpful in treating liver or gallbladder diseases, such as hepatitis, cirrhosis, or gallstones. Other conditions indirectly affected by liver function, such as endometriosis or side effects from chemotherapy, may also respond to these nutrients.

Choline, along with the B vitamins pantothenic acid and thiamin, may help treat heartburn as well.

ADDITIONAL BENEFITS
These two nerve-building nutrients may be useful for improving memory in those with Alzheimer's disease, preventing neural tube birth defects (spina bifida), boosting performance in endurance sports, and treating twitches and tics (tardive dyskinesia) caused by antipsychotic drugs. They have also been proposed as possible remedies against high cholesterol and even cancer. However, more studies are needed to define their role in these and other diseases.

▼ HOW TO TAKE IT

DOSAGE
Lecithin is usually given in a dosage of two 1,200 mg capsules twice a day. It can also be taken in a granular form: 1 teaspoon contains 19 grains, or 1,200 mg of lecithin.

Choline can be obtained from lecithin, although phosphatidylcholine (500 mg three times a day) or plain choline (500 mg three times a day) may be a better source. Choline can also be taken as part of a lipotropic combination product.

Lecithin and choline have no RDAs, although the scientific group that sets nutritional standards has established what's called an Adequate Intake (AI) for choline: 550 mg for men and 425 mg for women.

GUIDELINES FOR USE
• Lecithin and choline should be taken with meals to enhance absorption.

• Granular lecithin has a nutty taste and can be easily incorporated into your diet by sprinkling it over foods or mixing it into drinks.

FACTS & TIPS
■ Lecithin supplements vary widely in the amount of their active ingredient, phosphatidylcholine: It can range anywhere from 10% to 98%. In most cases, a higher concentration of phosphatidylcholine (and its extra cost) is not necessary.

■ Choline is so important for infant development that all FDA-approved infant formulas must contain this nutrient.

LATEST FINDINGS
■ Lack of choline shows up very quickly. Healthy adult men who were put on a strict 30-day choline-deficient diet displayed elevated liver enzymes, a clear indicator of liver problems. Supplementing their diet with lecithin restored their livers to their normal functioning.

■ It's a long way from rats to people, but a new study suggests a memory-enhancing effect for choline. Rats fed extra choline produced offspring that performed much better in memory and learning skills than those whose mothers were on a normal diet. Conversely, offspring of the rats deprived of choline did poorly on memory tests.

DID YOU KNOW?
Deficiencies in lecithin and choline are rare. Most Americans get enough of these nutrients in their daily diet—about 6 grams of lecithin and up to 1 gram of choline.

LICORICE *(Glycyrrhiza glabra)*

In ancient Greece, licorice once calmed coughs and soothed stomachs. In China, it's still thought to lengthen life. In fact, modern research has found that this versatile herb boosts immunity, fights viruses, treats ulcers, reduces inflammation, protects the liver, eases menopause, and applied topically, even relieves eczema.

COMMON USES

- Reduces symptoms of chronic fatigue and fibromyalgia.
- Helps digestive problems.
- Helps treat eczema.
- Promotes hepatitis recovery.
- Enhances immunity.
- Eases respiratory illnesses.
- May be useful for menstrual disorders and menopause.

FORMS

- Capsule/Tablet
- Liquid
- Wafer (DGL)
- Lozenge
- Cream
- Dried herb/Tea

▼ WHAT IT IS

One of the most extensively used and thoroughly studied herbal remedies, licorice has a long medicinal history. It was one of the first foods investigated by the National Cancer Institute's experimental food program.

Cultivated in Turkey and Greece, the licorice plant—a member of the pea family—is a tall shrub with bluish flowers. Its medicinal properties are in the root, or rhizome, which contains glycyrrhizin. Licorice is also a source of hundreds of other potentially beneficial substances, including plant estrogens and flavonoids.

Licorice root is made into capsules, tablets, liquids, and cream for therapeutic use. Because it has a sweet, musty taste, licorice root is frequently combined with other herbs to mask their bitterness.

Another form, DGL, or deglycyrrhizinated licorice, has had the glycyrrhizin removed; it is available in capsules and chewable wafers. The two types of licorice have different uses and effects on the body.

▼ WHAT IT DOES

The glycyrrhizin in licorice stimulates the adrenal glands to produce certain hormones, reduces inflammation, and increases the levels of interferon, a virus-fighting substance manufactured by the immune system. Other compounds in licorice are potent antioxidants and may also mimic the effects of estrogen in the body. DGL has a beneficial effect on the digestive tract.

MAJOR BENEFITS
Licorice is helpful for respiratory problems because it fights the viruses that attack the respiratory tract, relieves symptoms such as coughing and sore throat, and works to thin mucus.

Because of its action on the adrenal glands, licorice is often used by nutritionally oriented physicians to treat chronic fatigue syndrome, fibromyalgia, and other disorders affected by the body's levels of cortisol, the main adrenal hormone.

  ALERT

SIDE EFFECTS
- High doses of licorice root can raise blood pressure; they may also cause swelling, shortness of breath, and lethargy. DGL has no side effects.

CAUTION
- Do not exceed recommended dosages. Have your blood pressure monitored if you take licorice root longer than one month.

- Avoid licorice if you are pregnant or if you have heart, kidney, or liver disease or high blood pressure.

- Don't take licorice if you are on blood pressure medications, diuretics, hormone replacement therapy, or oral corticosteroids (i.e., prednisone).

- **Reminder:** If you have a medical condition, talk to your doctor before taking supplements.

The herb can also be taken for virtually any condition that involves inflammation. It's especially beneficial for hepatitis, combating inflammation in the liver and fighting the virus that often triggers the disease.

The DGL form does not work the same way licorice root does: DGL enhances the body's production of substances that coat the esophagus and stomach, protecting them from the corrosive effects of stomach acid. Therefore, DGL is helpful in cases of heartburn, ulcers, and inflammatory bowel disease.

In fact, in several studies, DGL was more effective than standard prescription anti-ulcer medications. It works only when mixed with saliva, however, which is why the chewable wafer form of DGL is preferred for digestive problems. These wafers can also speed the healing of canker sores.

ADDITIONAL BENEFITS

Licorice may be useful for menstrual problems and for menopause. Though glycyrrhizin inhibits the effect of the body's own estrogens, licorice's plant estrogens exert a mild estrogenic effect. A woman susceptible to PMS may find that taking licorice for 10 days leading up to her period eases some symptoms.

In addition, topical licorice creams soothe skin irritations, such as eczema.

▼ HOW TO TAKE IT

DOSAGE

For most disorders: Take licorice root three times a day in 200 mg pills (standardized to contain 22% glycyrrhizinic acid or glycyrrhizin) or as a liquid extract (½ to 1 teaspoon, or about 45 drops).
For heartburn and other digestive troubles: Chew two to four 380 mg DGL wafers three times a day.
For eczema: Apply cream to the affected area three or four times a day.

GUIDELINES FOR USE

• Licorice root supplements can be taken at any time of day.

• When using DGL, be sure to chew the wafers well and take them about 30 minutes before a meal.

• For sore throat, lozenges containing licorice work best.

LATEST FINDINGS

■ Preliminary studies in laboratory animals suggest a possible cancer-fighting role for licorice, particularly in preventing colon and breast cancer. Glycyrrhizin, its active ingredient, may be responsible for this effect because it can enhance immune-system activity. Plant estrogens found in the root may also be involved, at least as far as combating breast cancer is concerned.

■ Licorice may keep arteries clear and therefore help prevent heart disease, according to a recent study. Researchers found that taking 100 mg of licorice root a day was enough to minimize damage from LDL ("bad") cholesterol, a primary contributor to plaque formation. An active component in licorice was identified as glabridin, a substance present in supplements and standardized extracts, but not in licorice candy.

DID YOU KNOW?

Licorice candy in the United States is typically flavored with anise oil, not licorice root, and red licorice isn't really licorice at all. True licorice candy comes from Europe. Don't overindulge; it can elevate blood pressure just like licorice root does.

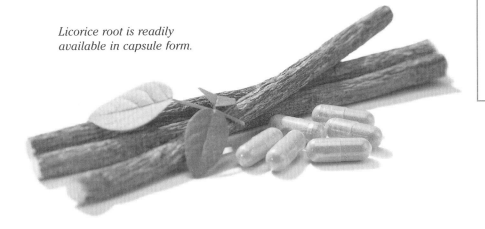

Licorice root is readily available in capsule form.

MAGNESIUM

Although little heralded, magnesium seems to be one of the most important health-promoting minerals. Studies suggest that besides enhancing approximately 300 enzyme-related processes in the body, magnesium may help prevent or combat many chronic diseases, ranging from asthma and fibromyalgia to heart disease.

COMMON USES

- Helps protect against heart disease and irregular heartbeat (arrhythmia).
- Eases fibromyalgia symptoms.
- Lowers high blood pressure.
- May help reduce the severity of asthma attacks.
- Improves symptoms of premenstrual syndrome (PMS).
- Aids in preventing the complications of diabetes.

FORMS

- Capsule
- Tablet
- Powder

▼ WHAT IT IS

The average person's body contains just an ounce of magnesium, but this small amount is vital to a number of bodily functions. Many people do not have adequate stores of magnesium, often because they rely too heavily on processed foods, which contain very little of this mineral. In addition, magnesium levels are easily depleted by stress, certain diseases or medications, and intense physical activity.

For this reason, nutritional supplements may be necessary for optimal health. They are available in several forms, including magnesium aspartate, magnesium carbonate, magnesium gluconate, magnesium oxide, and magnesium sulfate.

▼ WHAT IT DOES

One of the most versatile minerals, magnesium is involved in energy production, nerve function, muscle relaxation, and bone and tooth formation. In conjunction with potassium and calcium, magnesium regulates heart rhythm and clots blood; it also aids in the production and use of insulin.

PREVENTION

Recent research indicates that magnesium is beneficial for the prevention and treatment of heart disease. Studies show that the risk of dying of a heart attack is lower in areas with "hard" water, which contains high levels of magnesium. Some researchers speculate that if everyone drank hard water, the number of deaths from heart attacks might decline by 19%. Magnesium appears to lower blood pressure and has also been found to aid recovery after a heart attack by inhibiting blood clots, widening arteries, and normalizing dangerous arrhythmias.

Preliminary studies suggest that an adequate intake of magnesium may prevent type 2 (non-insulin-dependent) diabetes. Researchers at Johns Hopkins University measured magnesium levels in more than 12,000 people who did not have diabetes and tracked them for six years to see who developed the disease. Individuals with the lowest magnesium levels had a 94% greater chance of developing the disease than

ALERT

SIDE EFFECTS

- Some people develop nausea and diarrhea with magnesium supplements. If this happens to you, try reducing the dose or taking magnesium gluconate or magnesium sulfate, which are easier on the digestive tract.

CAUTION

- People with kidney disease should consult their physicians before taking magnesium supplements.

- Magnesium can make tetracycline antibiotics less effective. Consult your doctor before combining them.

- **Reminder:** If you have a medical condition, talk to your doctor before taking supplements.

those with the highest levels. (These study results, however, apply only to Caucasians; magnesium levels don't seem to affect diabetes in African-Americans.) Future studies are needed to see if magnesium supplements can prevent the disease.

ADDITIONAL BENEFITS
Because magnesium relaxes muscles, it's useful for sports injuries and fibromyalgia. It also seems to ease PMS and menstrual cramps, and may increase bone density in post-menopausal women, helping to stem the onset of osteoporosis.

In addition, magnesium expands airways, which aids in the treatment of asthma and bronchitis. Studies are inconclusive about magnesium's role in preventing or treating migraines, but one study says it may improve the effect of sumatriptan, a prescription drug used for migraines.

▼ HOW MUCH YOU NEED

The RDA for magnesium is 400 mg a day for men ages 19 to 30 (310 mg for women), and 420 mg a day for men ages 31 to 70 (320 mg for women). Higher doses of magnesium are required for disease prevention or treatment, as well as for women who take oral contraceptives.

IF YOU GET TOO LITTLE
Even moderate deficiencies can raise the risk of heart disease and diabetes. Severe deficiencies can result in irregular heartbeat, fatigue, muscle spasms, irritability, nervousness, and confusion.

IF YOU GET TOO MUCH
Magnesium can cause serious side effects—including muscle weakness,

lethargy, confusion, and difficulty breathing—if the body can't process high doses properly. Overdosing on magnesium, however, is rare because the kidneys are usually efficient at eliminating excess amounts.

▼ HOW TO TAKE IT

DOSAGE
For heart disease prevention: Take 400 mg a day.
For arrythmias, congestive heart failure, and asthma: Take 400 mg twice a day.
For fibromyalgia: Take 150 mg magnesium with 600 mg malic acid twice a day.
For high blood pressure: Take 400 to 800 mg a day.
For diabetes: Take 500 mg daily.

GUIDELINES FOR USE
• Magnesium is best absorbed when taken with each meal.

• Because magnesium can reduce the effectiveness of tetracycline antibiotics, take magnesium supplements one to three hours before or after the antibiotic medication.

▼ OTHER SOURCES

Good food sources of magnesium are whole grains, nuts, legumes, dark green leafy vegetables, and shellfish.

FACTS & TIPS

■ If you're taking magnesium supplements, take calcium supplements as well. Imbalances in the amounts of these two minerals can minimize the beneficial effects.

■ Research shows magnesium citrate is the form most readily absorbed by the body. Magnesium oxide may be the least expensive, but it's also the most poorly absorbed.

LATEST FINDINGS

■ A lack of magnesium can crimp a workout. In one study, women over age 50 needed more oxygen and had higher heart rates during exercise when magnesium levels were low.

■ Taking magnesium lowered blood pressure in a study of 60 men and women with hypertension. On average, systolic pressure (top number) dropped 2.7 points; diastolic pressure (bottom number) dropped 1.5 points. Declines of even a few points can reduce the risk of heart attack and stroke.

DID YOU KNOW?

You'd have to eat 3½ cups of wild rice to meet the RDA for a young man—400 mg of magnesium.

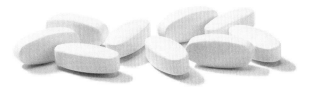

MELATONIN

Hailed by some proponents as a potent anti-aging hormone, melatonin has been credited with almost miraculous effects on a wide variety of ailments, including cancer, heart disease, and cataracts. It is probably most effective, however, as a natural sleep aid to ease insomnia and overcome jet lag.

COMMON USES

■ Relieves insomnia.

■ Promotes restful sleep, even during nighttime pain or stress-related disturbances in sleep.

■ Diminishes the effects and shortens the course of jet lag.

FORMS

■ Capsule

■ Tablet

■ Lozenge

■ Softgel

■ Liquid

▼ WHAT IT IS

First identified in 1958, this naturally occurring hormone is manufactured by the pineal gland, a pea-size organ deep within the brain. All humans and most animals secrete melatonin throughout their lives, with the highest levels occurring during childhood. As we age, however, the production of melatonin declines, leading some researchers to theorize that melatonin supplementation might benefit all older people.

Interestingly, natural melatonin levels vary widely: About 1% of the population have very low levels, and another 1% have levels 500 times above normal. There's no correlation, however, between these amounts and specific health concerns or sleep patterns.

▼ WHAT IT DOES

One of the main functions of melatonin is to regulate cycles of sleep and wakefulness. It does so by helping to set the brain's internal clock, creating what are known as circadian rhythms— the body's daily biorhythms that govern everything from sleeping and waking times to digestive functions and the release of a variety of hormones linked to reproduction and other body processes.

In order to produce melatonin, the body responds to light cues, making more melatonin when it's dark outside (production begins around dusk and peaks between 2 A.M. and 4 A.M.) and less during the day. This daily cyclical melatonin secretion is what tells the body when to sleep and when to awaken.

MAJOR BENEFITS

Melatonin may be most effective as a sleep aid. Various studies of both young and elderly adults indicate that in some people melatonin shortens the time needed to fall asleep and improves sleep quality by decreasing the number of times they awaken

 ALERT

SIDE EFFECTS

• No serious risks have been associated with 3 mg or less of melatonin, but long-term studies of six months or more have yet to be done.

• Melatonin can cause drowsiness within 30 minutes; its effect may last for several hours. Don't drive or handle heavy machinery during this time.

• Side effects can include headache, stomach upset, itchy skin, depression (transient), fast heartbeat, lethargy, or disorientation. Fuzzy thinking, vivid, unpleasant dreams, and even a worsening of insomnia may occur.

CAUTION

• Let your doctor know if you're taking melatonin. Adverse drug interactions have been reported in people taking common antidepressants (including Prozac or MAO inhibitors) or steroid or sedative drugs.

• Don't take melatonin if you are pregnant, breast-feeding, or trying to get pregnant (investigators are examining its effect on the menstrual cycle).

• Melatonin should not be taken by people with liver problems, depression, heart disease, or a neurologic disorder.

• **Reminder:** If you have a medical or psychiatric condition, talk to your doctor before taking supplements.

during the night. It may be beneficial when chronic pain or stress causes sleep disturbances.

Melatonin can also help restore normal sleep patterns in people who do night shift work or in those suffering from jet lag as a result of crossing time zones. Moreover, it works without producing the addictive effects of conventional sleep medications.

ADDITIONAL BENEFITS
Many other claims are made for melatonin. Interest in its possible anti-aging properties was sparked by an animal study in which nightly administration of the supplement to elderly mice prolonged their life by 25%. However, there have been no studies to date showing that melatonin supplementation delays aging in humans.

Some research suggests that it may boost the immune system. And it may be an even stronger antioxidant than vitamins C or E or beta-carotene, hunting down and destroying the naturally occurring, cell-damaging compounds called free radicals that can lead to heart disease, cataracts, and other age-related degenerative changes. More research is needed to determine if melatonin helps prevent these and other conditions.

Some studies suggest that when combined with certain cancer drugs, melatonin may help destroy malignant cells. Another study conducted in Holland in

1995 found that when taken in conjunction with birth control pills, melatonin has an estrogen-countering effect that may offer protection against some forms of breast cancer.

In addition, reports indicate that melatonin may reduce some of the nerve damage associated with both Alzheimer's and Parkinson's diseases. And a 1997 study from Italy revealed it may also have beneficial effects on the blood vessels and thus play a role in reducing the risk of stroke and heart attack. More research is needed to determine the effectiveness and long-term safety of melatonin for these and other uses.

▼ HOW TO TAKE IT

DOSAGE
For insomnia: Take 1 to 3 mg before bedtime.
For jet lag: Take a 3 mg dose on your day of travel, followed by 3 mg before bedtime for the first three or four nights at your final destination.
For shift work: Take a 3 mg dose at your desired bedtime (at 8 A.M., for example) after working a night shift.

GUIDELINES FOR USE
• To combat insomnia, stick to a precise schedule, taking supplements at the same time every evening.

• Begin with the lowest dose and increase it as needed.

SHOPPING HINTS
■ Most melatonin supplements (even those called "natural") are produced synthetically and are safe to buy. They're identical to natural human melatonin. However, be wary of melatonin products derived from animal glands; they may contain dangerous impurities.

LATEST FINDINGS
■ A study of 52 airline employees showed melatonin to be a very effective remedy against jet lag, significantly shortening the normal one-week adjustment period. Other studies with more than 400 people determined that the hormone reduces symptoms of jet lag by about 50%, on both eastward and westward flights.

■ Preliminary studies at the Oregon Health Sciences University in Portland found tiny doses of melatonin may be effective for wintertime blues. Depressed patients who received several doses of 0.1 mg of melatonin in the afternoon showed significant mood improvements, compared with those who received no melatonin or a larger single dose in the morning. Scientists speculate that small afternoon doses may better mimic the natural body processes, but caution against drawing conclusions.

DID YOU KNOW?
In Canada, Britain, France, and a number of other countries, melatonin is classified as a drug and is available by prescription only.

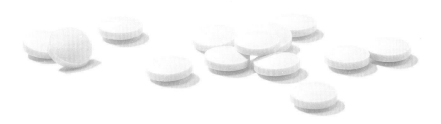

MILK THISTLE *(Silybum marianum)*

The medicinal use of milk thistle (widely called silymarin after its active ingredient) can be traced back thousands of years to the times of the Greeks and the Romans. Today, researchers have completed more than 300 scientific studies that attest to the benefits of this herb, particularly for treating liver-related ailments.

COMMON USES

■ Protects the liver from all kinds of toxins, including drugs, poisons, and chemicals.

■ Treats liver disorders, such as cirrhosis and hepatitis.

■ Reduces liver damage from drinking excessive alcohol.

■ Aids in the treatment and prevention of gallstones.

■ Helps clear psoriasis.

FORMS

■ Tablet

■ Capsule

■ Softgel

■ Liquid

▼ WHAT IT IS

Known by its botanical name, *Silybum marianum,* as well as by its principal active ingredient, silymarin, milk thistle is a member of the sunflower family. The purple flowers and milky white leaf veins of this herb, which early settlers brought from Europe to North America, are a common sight along the East Coast and in California; the plant also grows as a weed in other parts of the United States and around the world. It blooms from June through August, and the shiny black seeds used for medicinal purposes are collected at the end of summer.

▼ WHAT IT DOES

Milk thistle is one of the most extensively studied and documented herbs in use today. Scientific research continues to validate its healing powers, particularly for the treatment of liver-related disorders.

Most of its effectiveness stems from a complex of three liver-protecting compounds, collectively known as silymarin, which constitutes 4% to 6% of the ripe seeds.

MAJOR BENEFITS

Among the most important benefits of milk thistle is its ability to fortify the liver, which is one of the body's most important organs, second in size only to the skin. The liver processes nutrients, including fats and other foods. In addition, it breaks down and neutralizes, or detoxifies, many drugs, chemical pollutants, and alcohol.

Milk thistle helps enhance and even strengthen this vital organ by preventing the depletion of glutathione, an amino acid-like compound that is essential to the detoxifying process. What's more, studies show that milk thistle can increase glutathione concentration by up to 35%. This herb is also an effective gatekeeper, limiting the number of toxins that the liver processes at any given time.

Milk thistle is a powerful antioxidant as well. Even more potent than vitamins C and E, it helps prevent damage from highly reactive free-radical molecules. Furthermore, it promotes the regeneration of healthy, new liver cells, which

ALERT

SIDE EFFECTS
• Few side effects have been attributed to the use of milk thistle, which is considered one of the safest herbs on the market.

• In some people it may have a slight laxative effect for a day or two.

CAUTION
• Any liver disease requires careful medical evaluation and treatment under the supervision of a physician.

• **Reminder:** If you have a medical condition, talk to your doctor before taking supplements.

replace old and damaged ones. Milk thistle eases a range of serious liver ailments, including viral infections (hepatitis) and scarring of the liver (cirrhosis).

This herb is so potent that it's sometimes given in an injectable form in the emergency room to combat the life-threatening, liver-obliterating effects of poisonous mushrooms. In addition, because excessive alcohol depletes glutathione, milk thistle can aid in protecting the livers of alcoholics or those recovering from alcohol abuse.

ADDITIONAL BENEFITS
In cancer patients, milk thistle limits the potential for drug-induced damage to the liver after chemotherapy treatments, and it speeds recovery by hastening removal of toxic substances that can accumulate in the body.

The herb also reduces the inflammation and may slow the skin cell proliferation associated with psoriasis. It may be useful for endometriosis (the most common cause of infertility in women) because it helps the liver process the hormone estrogen, which at high levels can make pain and other symptoms worse.

Finally, milk thistle can be beneficial in preventing or treating gallstones because it improves the flow of bile, the cholesterol-laden digestive juice that travels from the liver through the gallbladder and into the intestine, where it helps to digest fats.

▼ HOW TO TAKE IT

DOSAGE
The recommended dose for milk thistle is up to 250 mg of standardized extract (containing 70% to 80% silymarin) or 1 teaspoon liquid extract three times a day.

Milk thistle is often combined with other herbs and nutrients, such as dandelion, choline, methionine, and inositol. This combination may be labeled "liver complex" or "lipotropic factors" ("lipotropic" refers to the formula's fat-metabolizing properties; it prevents the buildup of fatty substances in the liver). For proper dosage, follow package directions.

GUIDELINES FOR USE
• Milk thistle seems most effective when taken between meals.

• The benefits of milk thistle may be noticeable within a week or two, though long-term treatment is often needed for chronic conditions.

• No interactions between milk thistle and other medications have been noted to date.

SHOPPING HINTS
■ To be sure you're getting the proper dose, buy products made from standardized extracts that contain 70% to 80% silymarin, the active ingredient in milk thistle. You may also want preparations that contain milk thistle bound to phosphatidylcholine, a principal constituent of the natural fatty compound lecithin; studies show this combination may be better absorbed than regular milk thistle.

■ Be cautious about alcohol-based tinctures. Some formulas contain high amounts of alcohol, which can be bad for the liver if taken in large doses.

LATEST FINDINGS
■ Milk thistle may one day prove to be an important weapon in the battle against skin cancer. At Case Western Reserve University in Cleveland researchers found that when the active ingredient, silymarin, was applied to the skin of mice, 75% fewer skin tumors resulted following exposure to ultraviolet radiation. More studies are needed to see if it has a similar effect in humans.

DID YOU KNOW?
Milk thistle is not very soluble in water, so teas made from the seeds usually contain few of its liver-protecting ingredients.

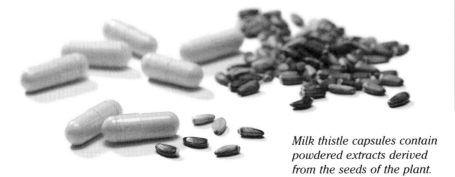

Milk thistle capsules contain powdered extracts derived from the seeds of the plant.

MUSHROOMS *(Shiitake, maitake, reishi, and PSK))*

Shiitake, reishi, and maitake are more than just exotic-sounding ingredients on a Japanese menu. In fact, they (along with an extract called PSK) are members of a special group of medicinal mushrooms that Asians have heralded for centuries as longevity tonics, immune-system boosters, and cancer fighters.

COMMON USES

- Build immunity.
- Help prevent cancer.
- Enhance cancer treatments.
- Alleviate bronchitis and sinusitis.
- Treat chronic fatigue syndrome.
- Help prevent heart disease.

FORMS

- Capsule
- Tablet
- Liquid
- Powder
- Tea
- Dried mushrooms
- Fresh mushrooms

▼ WHAT IT IS

For millennia, traditional Asian medicine has cherished certain mushrooms for their health-promoting effects. These include maitake *(Grifola frondosa)*, reishi *(Ganoderma lucidum)*, and shiitake *(Lentinus edodes)*. More recently, an extract from the mushroom *Coriolus versicolor*, called PSK, has also been found to be a potent cancer fighter.

Though other mushrooms—tree ear and oyster mushrooms, for instance—may also provide some health benefits, most of the attention and research have concentrated on the four types mentioned above.

These mushrooms are available as powders (in loose form for tea or in capsules or tablets) or as liquid extracts, which concentrate their potency. Dried reishi mushrooms and fresh and dried shiitake and maitake may be found in Asian groceries and some gourmet shops, but for therapeutic purposes, supplements are preferred. Maitake, reishi, and shiitake mushroom powders are sometimes combined in one capsule.

▼ WHAT IT DOES

Medicinal mushrooms have varied effects, including boosting the body's immune system, lowering cholesterol, acting as an anticoagulant, and playing a supporting role for other agents in the treatment of cancer.

MAJOR BENEFITS

Maitake and *Coriolus versicolor* are commonly used in Japan to strengthen the immune systems of people undergoing chemotherapy treatment for cancer. Studies have shown that maitake extracts increase the effectiveness of lower chemotherapy doses while protecting healthy cells from the damage such drugs can cause.

The Japanese have been employing the PSK extract from *Coriolus versicolor* as an adjunct to chemotherapy for many years. (In the United States, a similar product is labeled simply

ALERT

SIDE EFFECTS

- Shiitake, maitake, and reishi, as well as *Coriolus versicolor*, are all safe when used in appropriate doses.

- In rare cases, long-term use of reishi mushrooms—three to six months of daily use—can cause dry mouth, a skin rash and itchiness, an upset stomach, nosebleeds, or bloody stools. Stop taking reishi if symptoms arise.

CAUTION

- Pregnant or breast-feeding women should consult a physician before trying any of the mushrooms medicinally.

- People taking anticoagulant drugs (including a daily aspirin) should avoid reishi supplements because the mushrooms contain compounds that also "thin" the blood.

- **Reminder:** If you have a medical condition, talk to your doctor before taking supplements.

Coriolus versicolor extract.) Several studies have suggested that PSK can improve survival rates in people who have stomach, colon, or lung cancer, but more research is needed.

Medicinal mushrooms appear to boost the immune system, assisting the body in fighting disease-causing organisms. Some studies indicate they may be powerful enough to help people with HIV infection and AIDS (who have very weak immune systems).

For example, shiitake mushrooms contain a carbohydrate compound called lentinan, which promotes the body's production of T cells and other immune-system components. Laboratory studies show that *Coriolus versicolor* might be able to overpower HIV in the test tube; more research is needed, however, to see if it can do the same in the human body.

Other people with compromised immune systems—such as those with chronic fatigue syndrome—may benefit from medicinal mushrooms too.

ADDITIONAL BENEFITS
Traditionally, reishi (known to the Chinese as "spirit plants") are used to help people relax, making them suitable for reducing stress and fatigue. Reishi also contain anti-inflammatory compounds that are beneficial for

bronchitis and possibly for other respiratory ailments. In a Chinese study of 2,000 people with bronchitis, 60% to 90% of those given reishi tablets improved within two weeks.

Shiitake, maitake, and reishi may also help fight heart disease by reducing the tendency of blood to clot, lowering blood pressure, and possibly reducing cholesterol levels.

▼ HOW TO TAKE IT

DOSAGE
For immune-system support for cancer: Take 500 mg of reishi, 400 mg shiitake, and 200 mg maitake mushrooms three times a day, and/or 3,000 mg of *Coriolus versicolor*, divided into two doses, a day.
For heart disease or HIV/AIDS: Take 1,500 mg of reishi and 600 mg maitake daily.
For bronchitis or sinusitis: Take 1,500 mg of reishi and/or 600 mg maitake daily during the illness.

GUIDELINES FOR USE
• The effects of medicinal mushrooms aren't dramatic, and may need several months to appear.

• For best results, divide the supplements into two or three daily doses and take with or without food.

SHOPPING HINTS
■ *Coriolus versicolor* is available in limited supply in U.S. markets; this mushroom is expensive, costing about $1 per capsule (the recommended dose is five capsules a day). If you are undergoing chemotherapy treatment, you might deem the price worthwhile, or you can substitute less costly maitake mushrooms instead.

FACTS & TIPS
■ Don't forage for wild mushrooms, medicinal or culinary. It's too easy to mistake an edible fungus for a deadly one.

■ Powdered or dried mushrooms can be used to make an earthy-tasting tea or they can be added to soups. Dried mushrooms must simmer in liquid for at least 40 to 60 minutes to release their flavor and healing properties.

DID YOU KNOW?
The Japanese translation of maitake is "dancing mushroom," because if you find one, you dance for joy. Maitake mushrooms can weigh as much as a hundred pounds.

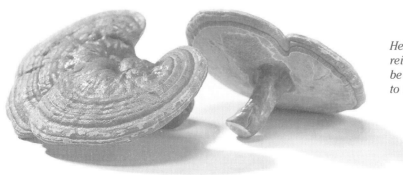

Helpful for stress, dried reishi mushrooms can be simmered in water to make a calming tea.

NETTLE *(Urtica dioica)*

The healing powers of this herb date to the third century B.C., when it was used to remove venom from snakebites. Today, scientists are confirming that nettle, with its stinging leaves, has a valuable role to play in treating hay fever and prostate symptoms, as well as in allieviating the pain and inflammation of gout.

COMMON USES

- Helps body remove excess fluid.
- Relieves allergy symptoms, particularly hay fever.
- Reduces inflammation.
- May ease prostate symptoms.
- Helps urinary tract infections.

FORMS

- Capsule
- Tincture
- Liquid
- Dried herb/Tea

▼ WHAT IT IS

Strange as it may sound, the original interest in using nettle for medicinal purposes probably was inspired by the plant's ability to irritate exposed skin. Nettle leaves are covered with tiny hairs—hollow needles actually—that sting and burn upon contact. This effect was believed to be beneficial for joint pain (stinging oneself with nettle is an old folk remedy for arthritis), and for centuries nettle leaf poultices were applied to draw toxins from the skin.

Also considered a nutritious food, nettle leaves taste like spinach. They are particularly high in iron and other minerals and are rich in carotenoids and vitamin C as well. (Opt for young shoots, which have no stingers.) The plant often grows up to five feet high in parts of the United States and Canada as well as in Europe.

▼ WHAT IT DOES

Stinging yourself with nettle leaves probably won't help your joint pain, but nettle tea applied as a compress or nettle supplements taken orally may relieve inflamed joints, especially in people with gout. In addition, when taken internally, nettle has diuretic and antihistamine properties.

MAJOR BENEFITS

As a diuretic, nettle helps the body rid itself of excess fluid, and it may be useful as an adjunct treatment for many disorders. People suffering from urinary tract infections, for example, may find that it promotes urination, which flushes infection-causing bacteria out of the body. Women who become bloated just before their period may experience some relief after taking nettle supplements.

The herb may also be of value in some cases of high blood pressure—which can partly be attributed to excess fluid in the body—but it should be used for this purpose only under the supervision of a doctor.

One of the tried-and-true benefits of nettle is its ability to control hay fever symptoms. Nasal congestion and watery eyes result when the body

  ALERT

SIDE EFFECTS

- Nettle is considered safe, with only a minimal risk of causing an allergic reaction. There have been some reports, however, that nettle root in particular may irritate the stomach, causing indigestion and diarrhea.

- Handling the fresh nettle plant itself can cause skin redness and irritation.

CAUTION

- Don't ever substitute nettle for a prescription medication for prostate problems without consulting your doctor.

- Nettle leaf preparations can cause complications in people with swelling (edema) related to heart or kidney problems.

Reminder: If you have a medical condition, talk to your doctor before taking supplements.

produces an inflammatory compound called histamine in response to pollen and other allergens.

Nettle is a good source of quercetin, a flavonoid that has been shown to inhibit the release of histamine. In one study of allergy sufferers, over half the participants rated nettle moderately to highly effective in reducing allergy symptoms when compared with a placebo.

ADDITIONAL BENEFITS
Nettle (specifically the root) may be suitable for men with an enlarged prostate not caused by cancer. This condition, called benign prostatic hyperplasia (BPH), occurs when the prostate enlarges and narrows the urethra (the tube that transports urine out of the bladder), making urination difficult. Nettle may aid in slowing prostate growth.

▼ HOW TO TAKE IT

DOSAGE
For urinary tract infections: Drink one cup of nettle leaf tea a day. Use 1 teaspoon of the dried herb per cup of very hot water.

For allergies: Take 250 mg nettle leaf standardized extract three times a day, as needed.
For gout: Take 250 mg nettle leaf three times a day. You can also apply a compress of nettle tea to painful joints.
For BPH: Use 250 mg nettle root standardized extract twice a day in combination with the herbs saw palmetto (160 mg twice a day) or pygeum africanum (100 mg twice a day).

GUIDELINES FOR USE
• In any of its forms, take nettle with food to minimize stomach upset.

• If you want to try the fresh leaves as a vegetable, keep in mind that the young shoots can be eaten raw, but older leaves (with mature, stinging hairs) must be cooked before eating to inactivate the stingers.

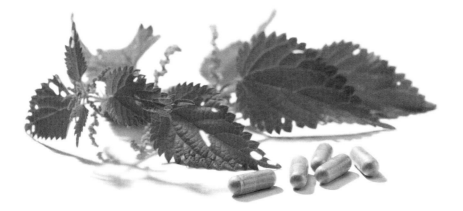

Supplements are a convenient way to get the diuretic and anti-histamine effects of nettle leaves.

SHOPPING HINTS
■ When buying nettle supplements, choose capsules that contain the freeze-dried herb, or an extract standardized to contain 1% plant silica, one of the active ingredients in nettle.

■ A nettle product must be made from the root of the nettle plant to be effective for prostate problems. When treating other ailments, select a product made from the leaf or other above-ground parts of the nettle plant.

LATEST FINDINGS
■ In a preliminary study, nettle helped arthritis patients reduce the amount of pain medication they needed and the drugs' side effects. Researchers found no difference in pain, stiffness, or the level of physical impairment between patients on 200 mg of the anti-inflammatory drug diclofenac (the brand name is Voltaren) and those taking 50 mg of the drug who also ate 2 ounces of nettle leaves each day. In previous studies, lowering the dose of diclofenac by just 25% lessened the drug's effectiveness in controlling symptoms of the disease.

■ In a recent study, nettle extract, when combined with pygeum africanum extract, appeared to block the hormonal changes believed to contribute to benign prostate enlargement.

NIACIN

This B vitamin has been in the limelight recently as a potent cholesterol-lowering agent because it rivals some prescription drugs in its effectiveness for this common condition. Beyond this, however, niacin in its various forms also shows promise in the prevention and treatment of depression, arthritis, and a host of other ailments.

COMMON USES

- Lowers cholesterol.
- May improve circulation.
- May ease symptoms of arthritis.
- May relieve depression.
- May prevent progression of type 1 diabetes.

FORMS

- Capsule
- Tablet

▼ WHAT IT IS

Also known as vitamin B_3, niacin is available as a supplement in three forms: nicotinic acid (or nicotinate), niacinamide, and inositol hexaniacinate (niacin bound to inositol, a member of the B-vitamin family). The body can also make niacin by converting the amino acid tryptophan—found in eggs, milk, and poultry—into the vitamin. About half of the niacin supplied by the average diet comes from the body's processing of tryptophan.

In supplement form, both nicotinic acid and niacinamide can satisfy your nutritional requirement for this B vitamin, but each of the three forms has its own specific role in treating disease.

▼ WHAT IT DOES

Niacin is needed to release energy from carbohydrates. It is also involved in controlling blood sugar, keeping the skin healthy, and maintaining the nervous and digestive systems.

PREVENTION

High doses of niacin raise HDL ("good") cholesterol, while lowering LDL ("bad") cholesterol and triglyceride levels. In fact, studies show that niacin may be more effective than prescription cholesterol-lowering drugs in reducing the risk of heart disease, mainly because it's one of the few agents that is known to boost HDL.

The cholesterol-lowering forms of niacin are nicotinic acid and inositol hexaniacinate. Although both are effective, inositol hexaniacinate is a safer form to use because it doesn't cause skin flushing and is less likely to cause liver damage.

ADDITIONAL BENEFITS

Niacin relaxes blood vessels, and so is useful for circulatory problems, such as intermittent claudication (a painful cramping in the calf caused by poor blood circulation that often occurs after walking) and Raynaud's disease (a disorder characterized by numbness and often pain in the hands or feet when exposed to cold). Inositol hexaniacinate is the preferred form to use for these conditions.

  ALERT

CAUTION

- Stick to recommended doses; excessive amounts of niacin can cause serious health problems.

- Consult your doctor before using any form of niacin if you have any of the following conditions: diabetes, low blood pressure, bleeding problems, glaucoma, gout, liver disease, or ulcers. All can be aggravated by niacin.

- Do not take therapeutic doses of any form of niacin if you also take cholesterol-lowering prescription drugs known as statins (including Fluvastatin, Pravastatin, Simvastatin).

- If you take a daily therapeutic dose of 1,000 mg or more of any form of niacin, be sure to see a doctor every three months to have your liver enzymes measured.

- **Reminder:** If you have a medical or psychiatric condition, talk to your doctor before taking supplements.

Niacin also helps foster healthy brain and nerve cells, and some evidence indicates that niacinamide can ease depression, anxiety, and insomnia.

Niacinamide seems to have an anti-inflammatory effect, which may benefit those with rheumatoid arthritis; it may also help repair cartilage, so it's potentially valuable for osteoarthritis.

High doses of niacinamide may reverse the development of type 1 diabetes—the form that typically appears before age 30—if this vitamin is given early enough. This therapy should be tried only with medical supervision.

▼ HOW MUCH YOU NEED

The RDA for niacin is 14 mg for women and 16 mg for men daily. But far higher doses are required to lower cholesterol and treat other disorders.

IF YOU GET TOO LITTLE
A slight niacin deficiency will cause patches of irritated skin, appetite loss, indigestion, and weakness. Severe deficiencies (practically nonexistent in industrialized countries) result in pellagra, a debilitating disease. Symptoms include a rash in areas exposed to sunlight, vomiting, a bright red tongue, fatigue, and memory loss.

IF YOU GET TOO MUCH
Therapeutic doses of nicotinic acid may cause stomach upset, flushing and itching of the skin, and liver damage (at high doses, niacinamide may also harm the liver). To prevent these side effects, substitute inositol hexaniacinate whenever possible: It eliminates skin flushing and greatly reduces the risk of liver damage. But if you're taking any form of niacin for long periods, have

your doctor do periodic blood tests to monitor your liver. Doses of inositol hexaniacinate higher than 2,000 mg a day may have a blood-thinning effect.

▼ HOW TO TAKE IT

DOSAGE
For lowering cholesterol, or treating Raynaud's disease or intermittent claudication: Take 500 to 1,000 mg of inositol hexaniacinate three times a day. When trying to reduce cholesterol, use the vitamin for two months; if your levels continue unchanged, stop taking the supplement.
For anxiety and depression: Take 50 mg of niacin a day; this is the dosage usually provided as part of a B-complex vitamin.
For insomnia: Take 500 mg niacinamide one hour before bedtime.
For arthritis: Take 1,000 mg niacinamide three times a day, but only under a doctor's supervision.

GUIDELINES FOR USE
• Take any form of niacin with meals or milk to decrease the likelihood of stomach upset.

▼ OTHER SOURCES

Niacin is found in foods high in protein, such as chicken, beef, fish, and nuts. Breads, cereals, and pasta are also enriched with niacin. Though they're low in niacin, milk and other dairy products, as well as eggs, are good sources of the vitamin because they're high in tryptophan.

FACTS & TIPS
■ Don't use over-the-counter timed-release niacin. It was developed to stop the skin flushing that high doses of nicotinic acid can cause, but studies show that it can damage the liver.

LATEST FINDINGS
■ In a study of niacin's effect on high cholesterol, participants who took niacin supplements had a 17% drop in LDL ("bad") cholesterol levels, a 16% rise in HDL ("good") cholesterol levels, and an 18% reduction in triglyceride levels.

■ The results of a study of niacinamide's effect on osteoarthritis showed that people who took the supplement for 12 weeks experienced more joint flexibility, less inflammation, and less need for anti-inflammatory drugs than those who were given a placebo.

DID YOU KNOW?
Pasta is often enriched with niacin. But you'd have to chow down 7 cups of cooked pasta to meet the RDA for this vitamin.

PAU D'ARCO *(Tabebuia impetiginosa)*

Rumored to have been prescribed by the ancient Incas to treat serious ailments, the herb pau d'arco, found in South American rain forests, has recently been investigated as a remedy for infectious diseases and cancer. Though its anticancer properties are debatable, pau d'arco may indeed combat a variety of infections.

COMMON USES

- Treats vaginal yeast infections.
- Helps get rid of warts.
- Reduces inflammation of the airways in bronchitis.
- May be useful in treating such immune-related disorders as asthma, eczema, psoriasis, and bacterial and viral infections.

FORMS

- Capsule
- Tablet
- Softgel
- Powder
- Liquid
- Dried herb/Tea

▼ WHAT IT IS

Pau d'arco is obtained from the inner bark of a tree—*Tabebuia impetiginosa*—indigenous to the rain forests of South America. Native tribes have taken advantage of its healing powers for centuries. Pau d'arco is also known as *lapacho, taheebo,* or *ipe roxo.* In the United States, however, it's always sold as pau d'arco.

The therapeutic ingredients in pau d'arco include a host of potent plant chemicals called naphthoquinones. Of these, a particular one called lapachol has been the most intensely studied by research investigators.

▼ WHAT IT DOES

Lapachol and other compounds in pau d'arco help destroy the microorganisms that can cause diseases and infections, ranging from malaria and the flu to yeast infections. Most people, however, are interested in the potential cancer-fighting properties of this herb.

MAJOR BENEFITS

Pau d'arco appears to combat bacteria, viruses, and fungi; reduce inflammation; and support the immune system. One of its best-documented uses is for vaginal yeast infections; herbalists often recommend a pau d'arco tea douche to restore the normal chemical environment of the vagina.

In capsule, tablet, tincture, or tea form, pau d'arco may be effective in strengthening immunity in people with chronic fatigue syndrome, HIV or AIDS, or chronic bronchitis. The herb's anti-inflammatory properties likewise benefit acute bronchitis, which involves inflammation of the respiratory passages, as well as muscle pain. And a tincture of pau d'arco applied directly to warts is useful in eradicating them.

ADDITIONAL BENEFITS

Pau d'arco's anticancer activity is subject to continuing debate. Because of the herb's traditional reputation as a cancer fighter, the National Cancer Institute (NCI) investigated it, identifying lapachol as its most active ingredient.

 ALERT

SIDE EFFECTS

- Whole-bark products are generally safe; they do not produce the side effects of high doses of lapachol. If pau d'arco tea or supplements cause stomach upset, take them with food.

- Unusual bruising or bleeding, pink urine, or severe nausea or vomiting are signs of an adverse reaction to pau d'arco. Stop taking the herb and call your doctor if they develop.

CAUTION

- Pregnant or lactating women should avoid pau d'arco.

- Take care if using pau d'arco with anticoagulant medications. The herb can amplify the drugs' blood-thinning actions, posing the risk of excessive bleeding and other problems. Consult your doctor for guidance.

- **Reminder:** If you have a medical condition, talk to your doctor before taking supplements.

In animal studies, pau d'arco showed promise in shrinking tumors, so the NCI began human trials using high doses of lapachol in the 1970s. Again, there was some evidence that lapachol was active in destroying cancer cells, but participants taking a therapeutic dose suffered serious side effects, including nausea, vomiting, and blood-clotting problems. As a result, research on lapachol and its source, pau d'arco, to treat cancer was abandoned.

Critics of this investigation believe that using therapeutic doses of pau d'arco—and not simply the isolated compound lapachol—would have produced similar benefits without the potentially danger-ous blood-thinning effects. It's likely that lapachol interferes with the action of vitamin K, needed for the blood to clot properly. Some researchers sug-gest that other compounds in pau d'arco supply some vitamin K, so that use of the whole herb would not inter-fere with blood clotting. Others think that combining lapachol with vitamin K supplements might make it possible for people to take doses of lapachol high enough to permit its potential anti-tumor action to be further studied without provoking a reaction.

Despite the controversy, many practi-tioners rely on the historical evidence of pau d'arco's anticancer action and often recommend it as a complement to conventional cancer treatment.

▼ HOW TO TAKE IT

DOSAGE
The typical daily dosage when using pau d'arco in capsule or tablet form is 250 mg twice a day; in liquid extract form it is 1 teaspoon twice a day.

This dose of pau d'arco is often rec-ommended for chronic fatigue syn-drome or HIV and AIDS in alternation with other immune-boosting herbs such as echinacea or goldenseal.

Pau d'arco is also commonly con-sumed as a tea in dried herb form. To make it, steep 2 or 3 teaspoons of pau d'arco in two cups of very hot water; drink the tea over the course of a day.

GUIDELINES FOR USE
• Many herbalists recommend using whole-bark products (not those that contain just lapachol). This is because they suspect that the herb's healing properties come from the interaction of the full range of plant chemicals in the bark.

• *For vaginal yeast infections:* Let pau d'arco tea cool to lukewarm before using it as a douche.

• *For warts:* Apply a compress soaked in pau d'arco liquid extract to the affected area at bedtime and leave it on all night. Repeat the treatment until the wart disappears.

SHOPPING HINTS
■ To be effective, pau d'arco prod-ucts must contain lapachol, which is found only in the bark of *Tabebuia impetiginosa,* not other *Tabebuia* species. One study examined the chemical makeup of 10 pau d'arco products and found that just one of them had any lapachol, the major active ingredient, indicating that either the wrong species or wrong part of the plant was used. The most effective pau d'arco products are those that are standardized to con-tain 2% to 7% lapachol, but these may be hard to find. Products that contain 3% naphthoquinones are of comparable quality.

FACTS & TIPS
■ Supplements are made from the inner bark of the pau d'arco tree, but in some parts of the world, the leaf of the tree is also valued for its therapeutic effects. In the Caribbean, for example, the leaf and bark have been used to relieve the acute pain of back-aches and toothaches.

■ Several South American tribes, including the Guarani and the Tupi, refer to the herb pau d'arco as "*tajy,*" which means "to have strength and vigor."

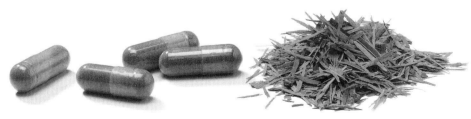

Pau d'arco can be taken as a supplement or brewed as a tea.

PEPPERMINT *(Mentha piperita)*

For centuries this powerfully aromatic herb has provided relief for indigestion, colds, and headache. Today, medicinal peppermint is most prized for its ability to soothe the digestive tract, easing indigestion, irritable bowel syndrome, and other complaints. It's also useful for relieving muscle aches and freshening stale breath.

COMMON USES

■ Relieves heartburn, nausea, and indigestion; helps dissolve gallstones.

■ Eases symptoms of diverticulosis and irritable bowel syndrome.

■ Sweetens the breath.

■ Soothes muscle aches.

■ Eases coughs and congestion.

FORMS

■ Capsule

■ Oil

■ Ointment/Cream

■ Tincture/Liquid

■ Dried or fresh herb/Tea

▼ WHAT IT IS

Peppermint is cultivated worldwide for use as a flavoring agent and an herbal medicine. A natural hybrid of spearmint and water mint, peppermint has square stems and oval, pointed dark green or purple leaves and lilac flowers. For medicinal purposes, the plant's leaves and stems are harvested just before the flowers bloom in summer.

The major active ingredient of peppermint is its volatile oil, which is made up of more than 40 different compounds. The oil's therapeutic effect comes mainly from menthol (35% to 55% of the oil), menthone (15% to 30%), and menthyl acetate (3% to 10%). Medicinal peppermint oil is made by steam-distilling the parts of the plant that grow above the ground.

▼ WHAT IT DOES

Particularly effective in treating digestive disorders, peppermint relieves cramps and relaxes intestinal muscles. It freshens the breath and may clear up nasal congestion as well.

MAJOR BENEFITS

Peppermint oil relaxes the muscles of the digestive tract, helping to relieve intestinal cramping and gas. Its antispasmodic effect also makes it useful for alleviating the symptoms of irritable bowel syndrome, a common disorder characterized by abdominal pain, alternating bouts of constipation and diarrhea, and indigestion.

The menthol in peppermint aids digestion because it stimulates the flow of natural digestive juices and bile. This explains why peppermint oil is often included in over-the-counter antacids.

Several studies indicate that the menthol in peppermint oil assists in dissolving gallstones as well, providing a possible alternative to surgery. Consult your doctor before trying the oil for this purpose. You can also put the oil directly on your tongue; it provides a minty antidote to bad breath.

  ALERT

SIDE EFFECTS

• Peppermint leaves in recommended doses generally produce no side effects. Rarely, peppermint oil capsules cause a skin rash and/or heartburn.

• Topical peppermint oil can cause allergic skin rashes, especially if you're applying heat as well. If side effects occur, stop using the herb.

CAUTION

• Because peppermint oil relaxes gastrointestinal muscles, it may aggravate the symptoms of a hiatal hernia.

• Avoid large doses of peppermint oil during pregnancy.

• Peppermint oil should not be applied to the nostrils or chest of infants and children under age 5 because it can cause a choking sensation.

• Never ingest pure menthol, a major ingredient in peppermint oil; as little as 1 teaspoon (2 grams) can cause a severe reaction.

• **Reminder:** If you have a medical condition, talk to your doctor before taking supplements.

As a tea or oil, peppermint serves as a mild anesthetic to the stomach's mucous lining, which helps reduce nausea and motion sickness. The tea may ease symptoms of diverticulosis as well, including gas and bloating.

ADDITIONAL BENEFITS

When rubbed on the skin, peppermint oil relieves pain by stimulating the nerves that perceive cold while muting those that sense pain, making it a welcome remedy for aching muscles.

Findings are contradictory concerning peppermint's historical use in the treatment of colds and coughs. Some tests show the aromatic plant has no effect. But Commission E, a German health board recognized as an authority on the scientific investigation of herbs, found that peppermint was an effective decongestant that reduced inflammation of the nasal passageways. In addition, many people with colds report that inhaling peppermint's menthol enables them to breathe more easily. Drinking warm peppermint tea also may offer relief from the bronchial constriction of asthma.

▼ HOW TO TAKE IT

DOSAGE

For the treatment of irritable bowel syndrome, nausea, and gallstones: Try enteric-coated capsules containing peppermint oil because they release peppermint oil where it's

The oil from peppermint leaves helps relieve many digestive complaints.

most needed—in the small and large intestine rather than in the stomach. Take one or two capsules (containing 0.2 ml of oil per capsule) two or three times a day, between meals.

To freshen the breath: Place a few drops of peppermint oil on the tongue.

To relieve gas and calm the stomach: Make a tea by steeping 1 or 2 teaspoons of dried peppermint leaves in a cup of very hot water for between 5 and 10 minutes; be sure to cover the cup to keep the volatile oil from escaping.

For congestion: Drink up to four cups of peppermint tea a day.

For pain relief: Add a few drops of peppermint oil to ½ ounce of a neutral oil. Apply to the affected areas up to four times daily.

GUIDELINES FOR USE

• Take enteric-coated capsules between meals.

• If you prefer peppermint tea, drink a cup three or four times a day, right after or between meals.

• Apply peppermint oil or ointments containing menthol no more than three or four times daily.

• To use peppermint tincture, put 10 to 20 drops of the tincture in a glass of water and drink; to take liquid extract, put ½ to 1 teaspoon of the extract in a glass of water and drink.

FACTS & TIPS

■ Peppermint oil appears in more commercial products than any other herb. Included in antacids for its therapeutic effects, the oil is also added to toothpaste and mouthwash for the freshness it imparts.

■ Many people confuse peppermint with another popular mint: spearmint. Unlike peppermint, however, spearmint contains no menthol to aid digestion.

LATEST FINDINGS

■ In a study conducted at the Taichung Veterans General Hospital in Taiwan, the vast majority of patients with irritable bowel syndrome who took enteric-coated peppermint oil capsules 15 to 30 minutes before every meal reported significant relief. Abdominal pain was reduced or disappeared entirely, and patients had less bloating, less frequent stools, and less stomach rumbling and flatulence than usual.

■ Researchers at the University of Kiel in Germany studied the effect of peppermint oil on headaches. They found that applying a mixture of peppermint and eucalyptus oils and ethanol to the forehead and temples significantly reduced pain.

DID YOU KNOW?

Peppermint's stomach-settling ability makes it a popular ingredient in after-dinner mints, though few confections contain much peppermint oil.

PHOSPHORUS

If you compiled a list of nutrients the body could not live without, phosphorus would doubtless be near the top. Although the main function of phosphorus is building strong bones and teeth (in conjunction with calcium), this mineral is needed by virtually every cell. Fortunately, the chance of a phosphorus deficiency is very small.

COMMON USES

- Builds strong bones and maintains skeletal integrity.
- Helps form tooth enamel and strengthens teeth.

FORMS

- Capsule
- Tablet
- Powder
- Liquid

▼ WHAT IT IS

Phosphorus is the second most abundant mineral in the body (after calcium), and up to one and a half pounds of it are found in the average person. Although 85% of this mineral is concentrated in the bones and teeth, the rest is distributed in the blood and in various organs, including the heart, kidneys, brain, and muscles.

Phosphorus interacts with a variety of other nutrients, but its most constant companion is calcium. In the bones, the ratio of calcium to phosphorus is around 2:1. In other tissues, however, the amount of phosphorus is higher.

▼ WHAT IT DOES

There is hardly a biological or cellular process that does not, directly or indirectly, involve phosphorus. In some instances, the mineral works to protect cells, strengthening the membranes that surround them. In other cases, it acts as a kind of biological escort, assisting a variety of nutrients, hormones, and chemicals in doing their jobs. There's also evidence that phosphorus helps activate the B vitamins, enabling them to provide all their benefits.

MAJOR BENEFITS

One of phosphorus's most important functions is to team up with calcium to build bones and aid in maintaining a healthy, strong skeleton. The calcium-phosphorus partnership is also crucial for strengthening the teeth and helping to keep them strong.

In addition, phosphorus joins with fats in the blood to make compounds called phospholipids, which, in turn, play structural and metabolic roles in cell membranes throughout the body. Furthermore, without phosphorus, the body could not convert the proteins, carbohydrates, and fats it absorbs from food into energy.

The mineral is needed to create the molecule known as adenosine triphosphate, or ATP, which acts like a tiny battery charger, supplying vital energy to every cell in the body.

ADDITIONAL BENEFITS

Phosphorus serves as a cell-to-cell messenger. In this capacity, it helps

 ALERT

CAUTION

- The greatest risk associated with phosphorus may be getting too much, which some experts caution may lead to a calcium deficiency. Never take phosphorus supplements without discussing it with your doctor first.

- In the rare instance of a phosphorus deficiency—such as from kidney or digestive disease or a severe burn—phosphorus supplementation must be medically supervised.

- **Reminder:** If you have a medical condition, talk to your doctor before taking supplements.

the coordination of such body processes as muscle contraction, the transmission of nerve impulses from the brain to the body, and the secretion of hormones. An adequate phosphorus supply may therefore enhance your physical performance and be effective in fighting fatigue.

In addition, the mineral is necessary for maintaining the pH (the acid-base balance) of the blood and for manufacturing DNA and RNA, the basic components of our genetic makeup.

▼ HOW MUCH YOU NEED

Because phosphorus is found in so many foods, the need for supplements is virtually nonexistent. The RDA for phosphorus in men and women is the same, 700 mg daily. In the past, many nutritionists recommended that phosphorus and calcium be taken in a 1:1 ratio, but recently, experts have advised that this ratio has little practical benefit. Most people today consume more phosphorus than calcium in their diets.

IF YOU GET TOO LITTLE
Although rare, a deficiency of phosphorus can lead to fragile bones and teeth, fatigue, weakness, a loss of appetite, joint pain and stiffness, and an increased susceptibility to infection. A mild deficiency may produce a modest decrease in energy.

IF YOU GET TOO MUCH
There are no immediate adverse effects from getting too much phosphorus.

However, some experts caution that over the long term, excessive phosphorus intake may inhibit calcium absorption, though it's uncertain whether this can result in a calcium deficiency that threatens bone health.

▼ HOW TO TAKE IT

DOSAGE
Most people get all the phosphorus they require through their everyday diet. In addition, a small amount of phosphorus may be included in daily multivitamin and mineral supplements.

If you have a medical condition that depletes this mineral, such as a bowel ailment or failing kidneys, your doctor will prescribe an appropriate dose.

GUIDELINES FOR USE
• Never take individual phosphorus supplements without being under a doctor's supervision.

▼ OTHER SOURCES

High-protein foods, such as meat, fish, poultry, and dairy products, contain a lot of phosphorus. It is also used as an additive in many processed foods. Soft drinks, particularly colas, often have large amounts too.

Phosphorus is present in grain products as well, although whole grain breads and cereals may include ingredients that partially reduce the absorption of this mineral.

FACTS & TIPS
■ The aluminum present in some antacids can diminish phosphorus levels in the body. If you habitually take antacids, talk to your doctor about your particular need for phosphorus supplements.

LATEST FINDINGS
■ One study showed teenage girls who regularly consume great amounts of phosphorus-rich cola beverages are at greater risk for bone fractures than non-soda drinkers. Experts disagree, however, on whether it's the phosphorus at work. They point out that soda drinkers are much less likely to drink milk—and therefore do not get enough of the bone-building mineral calcium in their diets.

■ Swiss researchers report that phosphorus supplementation may be especially beneficial for burn victims, who were found to have low phosphorus levels within a week of suffering severe burns. Supplements may be necessary to restore patients to full health following a major burn injury.

DID YOU KNOW?
The average American diet contains between 1,000 and 1,500 mg of phosphorus daily, well above the RDA for this mineral.

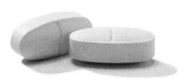

POTASSIUM

You're probably careful not to eat too much sodium (salt), especially if you're watching your blood pressure. You might also want to focus your efforts, however, on getting more potassium. For some people, stocking up on this mineral may be as important to blood pressure control as limiting the sodium they eat.

COMMON USES

 Helps lower blood pressure.

 May prevent high blood pressure, heart disease, and stroke.

FORMS

 Tablet

 Liquid

 Powder

▼ WHAT IT IS

The third most abundant mineral in the body after calcium and phosphorus, potassium is an electrolyte—a substance that takes on a positive or negative charge when dissolved in the watery medium of the bloodstream. Sodium and chloride are electrolytes too, and the body needs a balance of these minerals to perform a host of essential functions. Almost all the potassium in the body is found inside the cells.

▼ WHAT IT DOES

Along with the other electrolytes, potassium is used to conduct nerve impulses, initiate muscle contractions, and regulate heartbeat and blood pressure. It controls the amount of fluid inside the cells, and sodium regulates the amount outside, so the two minerals work in concert to balance fluid levels in the body.

Potassium also enables the body to convert blood sugar (glucose)—its primary fuel—into a stored form of energy (glycogen) that's held in reserve by the muscles and liver.

PREVENTION

Study after study has shown that people who get plenty of potassium in their diets have lower blood pressure than those who get very little. This effect holds true even when sodium intake remains high (though reducing sodium produces better results).

In one study, 54 people on medication for high blood pressure were divided into two groups. Half followed their regular diet; the other half added three to six servings of potassium-rich foods a day. After a year, 81% of those getting extra potassium were able to reduce their drug dosages significantly, compared with only 29% of the individuals following their regular diets.

ADDITIONAL BENEFITS

Through its effects on blood pressure, potassium may also decrease the risk of heart disease and stroke. In one study, a group of people with hypertension who ate one serving of a food high in potassium every day reduced their risk of fatal stroke by 40%. A 12-year investigation found that men who got the least amount of potassium were two and a half times more likely to die from a stroke than men who consumed the most; for women with

ALERT

CAUTION

• Do not take potassium supplements without consulting your doctor if you have kidney disease, are taking corticosteriods, or are using any medication for high blood pressure or heart disease.

• **Reminder:** If you have a medical condition, talk to your doctor before taking supplements.

a low potassium intake, the risk of fatal stroke was nearly five times greater.

▼ HOW MUCH YOU NEED

There is no RDA for potassium, but most experts recommend 2,000 to 3,000 mg a day. More may be needed to control blood pressure.

IF YOU GET TOO LITTLE
Potassium is found in a wide variety of foods, so it is practically impossible not to get enough of this mineral to perform the basic body functions. But a serious deficiency can occur if an individual is taking a potent diuretic (a drug that reduces fluid levels in the body) or is suffering from an extreme case of diarrhea or vomiting. The first sign of deficiency is muscle weakness and nausea. If potassium is not replaced, low levels could lead to heart failure.

IF YOU GET TOO MUCH
Potassium toxicity is highly unlikely because most people can safely consume up to 18 grams a day. Toxicity usually occurs only if an individual has a kidney disorder or takes too many potassium supplements. Signs of potassium overload include muscle fatigue and an irregular heartbeat. Even in small doses, potassium supplements may cause stomach irritation and nausea.

▼ HOW TO TAKE IT

DOSAGE
Most people don't need potassium supplements unless they are taking certain diuretic medications. Try to get sufficient potassium in your daily diet; if you want extra insurance, take no more than 500 mg of potassium in supplement form a day.

People who use ACE inhibitors (such as captopril or enalapril) for high blood pressure or angina and those who have kidney disease should not take potassium supplements at all.

GUIDELINES FOR USE
• If you use potassium supplements, take them with food to decrease stomach irritation.

• Many nutritionally oriented doctors believe you really don't need to take potassium supplements unless specifically advised to do so by your healthcare practitioner. Potassium-rich foods are a better option for those who wish to maintain good health.

▼ OTHER SOURCES

Fresh fruits and vegetables—such as bananas, oranges and orange juice, and potatoes—are very high in potassium. Meats, poultry, milk, and yogurt are also good sources.

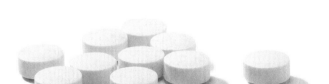

FACTS & TIPS
■ Microwave or steam vegetables whenever possible—boiling them decreases their potassium content. For example, boiled potatoes lose 50% of their potassium; steamed potatoes lose less than 6%.

■ By law, over-the-counter potassium supplements cannot contain more than 99 mg per pill (this includes multivitamin and mineral preparations). If you think you need potassium supplements, talk to your doctor about higher-dose pills available by prescription.

LATEST FINDINGS
■ An analysis of the results of 33 studies confirms that potassium has a positive impact on blood pressure. People with normal blood pressure who added 2,340 mg of potassium a day—from foods, supplements, or a combination—to their diets had an average drop of 2 points in systolic blood pressure (the upper reading) and 1 point in diastolic pressure (the lower). If this sounds insignificant, consider that even these small changes reduce the chance of developing hypertension by 25%. The extra potassium produced even greater benefits—a 4.4 point drop in systolic pressure and a 2.5 point drop in diastolic—in people who already had high blood pressure.

DID YOU KNOW?
A large navel orange has 250 mg of potassium, about a quarter of what most people consume daily.

PSYLLIUM *(Plantago psyllium, P. ovata)*

These tiny plant seeds are so rich in fiber that they've been prescribed for constipation and a wide range of other digestive ailments for more than 500 years. Now, new research is finding that psyllium offers an added benefit as well: The seeds appear to lower blood cholesterol levels both safely and effectively.

COMMON USES

- Relieves constipation, diarrhea.
- Treats diverticular disease and irritable bowel syndrome.
- Helps prevent gallstones.
- Reduces hemorrhoid pain.
- May lower cholesterol.
- Facilitates weight loss.

FORMS

- Powder
- Capsule
- Wafer

▼ WHAT IT IS

Odorless and nearly tasteless, psyllium comes from the small, reddish brown to black seeds of the *Plantago psyllium* plant. Also known as the plantain, it should not be confused with the edible bananalike fruit of the same name *(Musa paradisiaca)* or with the herb plantain *(Plantago lanceolata)* sometimes recommended for coughs.

Plantago psyllium grows as a weed in numerous places around the world and it is commercially cultivated in Spain, France, India, Pakistan, and other countries.

Various species of the plant are used in herbal medicine, most commonly the seeds of *Plantago psyllium* and *P. ovata*. These seeds, so tiny that they are sometimes called "flea seeds," are generally dried, ground, and sold in powder, capsule, or chewable tablet (wafer) form. Psyllium is sometimes added to breakfast cereals.

▼ WHAT IT DOES

When mixed with water, the fibrous, mucilage-covered husks of psyllium seeds form a gel-like mass that absorbs excess water from the intestines and creates larger, softer stools. Psyllium helps to lower cholesterol by binding to cholesterol-rich bile in the digestive tract, causing the body to draw cholesterol from the bloodstream.

As an inexpensive source of soluble fiber (the kind of fiber that blends with water), it's particularly suitable for those people who don't eat enough fiber-rich foods, such as whole grains (oats are particularly rich in soluble fiber), beans, fruits, and vegetables.

MAJOR BENEFITS

Psyllium can help normalize bowel function in a wide variety of disorders, including constipation, diarrhea, diverticulosis, hemorrhoids, and irritable bowel syndrome. It does so by a single mechanism: absorbing water, which lends bulk to stools. In the case of

 ▦ ALERT ▦

SIDE EFFECTS

- Psyllium can cause temporary bloating and increased flatulence because it supplies fiber. Avoid these problems by slowly increasing psyllium intake over several days.

- Don't exceed recommended doses; taking larger quantities of psyllium can reduce your body's ability to absorb certain minerals.

CAUTION

- Always take psyllium with plenty of liquid. Without lots of fluid, it is possible to develop an intestinal blockage, which can cause severe, painful constipation.

- Allergic reactions, though rare, can be life-threatening; if you have trouble swallowing or breathing, seek immediate medical help.

- Some people are allergic to psyllium. Reactions are often quick, marked by a rash, itching, and in severe cases, difficulty breathing or swallowing. Get immediate medical help.

- **Reminder:** If you have a medical condition, talk to your doctor before taking supplements.

constipation, the added water and bulk help soften stools, making them easier to pass.

Although psyllium doesn't cure hemorrhoids, passing softer stools reduces irritation in the tender area. In one study, 84% of hemorrhoid sufferers receiving a supplement containing psyllium reported less bleeding and pain. Psyllium has also been reported to have a soothing effect on those with irritable bowel syndrome.

In people with diverticular disease—in which small pockets in the intestine's lining trap fecal particles and become susceptible to infection—psyllium bulks the stools and speeds their passage through the intestine, helping to alleviate the problem. And psyllium's ability to absorb large amounts of excess water from loose stools is an effective treatment for diarrhea.

ADDITIONAL BENEFITS

Although psyllium has been used for constipation for centuries, only in the 1980s did scientists discover another benefit: This herb reliably lowers levels of blood cholesterol, especially the "bad" LDL cholesterol that can stick to artery walls and lead to heart disease. In several studies of men and women with high cholesterol levels, taking in 10 grams or more of psyllium daily for six weeks or longer lowered LDL from 6% to 20% more than consuming a low-fat diet did. Sometimes, simply adding psyllium to your diet is enough to eliminate the need for cholesterol-lowering medications.

This fiber source may also play a role in weight-loss programs. By absorbing water, psyllium fills the stomach, providing a sense of fullness. It also delays the emptying of food from the stomach, thus extending the length of time you feel full.

In a small British study, women who took psyllium with water three hours before they ate consumed less fat and fewer calories during the meal itself. Whether this effect persists and leads to long-term weight loss, however, is unknown. And psyllium can help stabilize levels of glucose (sugar) in the blood, which may control food cravings.

▼ HOW TO TAKE IT

DOSAGE
The dose of a psyllium product depends on the concentration of soluble fiber in the product and can range from 1 teaspoon three times a day to 3 tablespoons three times a day. Read the package carefully to determine the correct dose of your psyllium product.

GUIDELINES FOR USE
• Relief of constipation usually occurs in 12 to 24 hours, although it can take as long as three days.

• Because psyllium absorbs water, always consume it with large amounts of fluid. Dissolve psyllium powder in water (or juice), drink it, and then drink another glass of water or juice. In addition to this fluid, drink six to eight glasses of water a day.

• Take psyllium two hours or more after taking medications or other supplements so that it doesn't inhibit the absorption of the drugs.

• If you are pregnant, have diabetes, or have an obstructed bowel (possibly signaled by persistent constipation or abdominal pain), check with a doctor before using psyllium.

FACTS & TIPS
■ In 1998, the Food and Drug Administration (FDA) allowed breakfast cereals containing psyllium to claim that they reduce the risk of heart disease as part of a diet low in saturated fat and cholesterol. To qualify, a cereal must contain 1.7 grams of soluble fiber from psyllium per serving. Four servings a day deliver 7 grams of soluble fiber, enough to lower blood cholesterol significantly. Combining a psyllium-enriched cereal with a whole-oat cereal may be an even more effective cholesterol-lowering strategy.

LATEST FINDINGS
■ Not only may psyllium aid in weight loss by suppressing appetite, but it may also prevent gallstones. A Mexican study of obese patients on very low calorie diet, which increases the risk for gallstones, found that psyllium helped avert this sometimes acutely painful condition.

■ Psyllium lowers cholesterol even in youngsters. In a study of 25 children ages 6 to 18 who had high cholesterol, adding a cereal containing psyllium to a low-fat diet reduced harmful LDL cholesterol by an additional 7%.

DID YOU KNOW?
In Europe during the Middle Ages, Arab physicians sold a constipation remedy called diagridium. Psyllium was one of its main ingredients.

RIBOFLAVIN

For decades riboflavin, also known as vitamin B_2, was largely overlooked. But recently, thanks to exciting new research, this vitamin has been praised for its potential healing powers, including battling painful migraines, preventing sight-robbing cataracts, treating nerve-related conditions, healing skin blemishes—and much more.

COMMON USES

■ Prevents or delays the onset of cataracts.

■ Reduces the frequency and severity of migraines.

■ Improves skin blemishes caused by rosacea.

FORMS

■ Tablet

■ Capsule

■ Liquid

■ Powder

▼ WHAT IT IS

Looking through a microscope in 1879, scientists discovered a fluorescent yellow-green substance in milk, but not until 1933 was the substance identified as riboflavin. This water-soluble vitamin is part of the B-complex family, which is involved in transforming protein, fats, and carbohydrates into fuel for the body.

Found naturally in many foods, riboflavin is also added to fortified breads and cereals. It is easily destroyed when exposed to light. Inadequate riboflavin intake often accompanies B-vitamin deficiencies, which are a common problem in the elderly and alcoholics. Riboflavin is available as a single supplement, in combination with other B vitamins (vitamin B complex), or as part of a multivitamin.

▼ WHAT IT DOES

The body depends on riboflavin for a wide range of functions. It plays a vital role in the production of thyroid hormone, which speeds up metabolism and helps assure a steady supply of energy. Riboflavin also aids the body in producing infection-fighting immune cells; it works in conjunction with iron to manufacture red blood cells, which transport oxygen to all the cells in the body. In addition, it converts vitamins B_6 and niacin into active forms so that they can do their work.

Riboflavin produces substances that assist powerful antioxidants, such as vitamin E, in protecting cells against damage from the naturally occurring, highly reactive molecules known as free radicals.

Riboflavin is essential for tissue maintenance and repair—the body uses extra amounts to speed the healing of wounds after surgery, burns, and other injuries. The vitamin is also necessary to maintain the function of the eye and may be important for healthy nerves too.

PREVENTION

By boosting antioxidant activity, riboflavin protects many body tissues—particularly the lens of the eye. It may therefore help prevent the formation of cataracts, the milky opacities in the lens that impair the vision of so many older people. Ophthalmologists urge everyone, especially those with a family history of this eye disorder, to get an adequate and steady supply of riboflavin throughout their lives.

ALERT

CAUTION

• Consult your doctor if you are taking oral contraceptives, antibiotics, or psychiatric drugs, which can affect riboflavin needs.

• **Reminder:** If you have a medical or psychiatric condition, talk to your doctor before taking supplements.

The vitamin has also been shown to be highly effective in reducing the frequency and severity of migraine headaches. Migraine sufferers are believed to have reduced energy reserves in the brain, and riboflavin may prevent attacks by increasing the energy supply to brain cells.

ADDITIONAL BENEFITS

Riboflavin has proved valuable in treating skin disorders, including rosacea, which causes facial flushing and skin pustules in many adults.

In combination with other B vitamins, including vitamin B_6 and niacin, riboflavin may help protect against a broad range of nerve and other ailments, including Alzheimer's disease, epilepsy, numbness and tingling, and multiple sclerosis, as well as anxiety, stress, and even fatigue. Some doctors will prescribe extra riboflavin supplementation to treat sickle-cell anemia, because many patients with this condition have a riboflavin deficiency.

▼ HOW MUCH YOU NEED

The daily RDA for riboflavin is 1.3 mg for men and 1.1 mg for women. These amounts simply prevent general deficiencies; larger doses are usually prescribed for specific conditions.

IF YOU GET TOO LITTLE

Classic deficiency symptoms include cracking and sores in the corner of the mouth and increased sensitivity to light, with tearing, burning, and itchy eyes. The skin around the nose, eyebrows, and earlobes may peel, and there may be a skin rash in the groin area. A low red blood cell count (or anemia), resulting in fatigue, can also sometimes occur.

IF YOU GET TOO MUCH

Excess riboflavin isn't dangerous because the body excretes any extra in the urine. However, high intakes of this vitamin can turn the urine bright yellow—which is a harmless but somewhat unsettling side effect.

▼ HOW TO TAKE IT

DOSAGE

For cataract prevention: The usual dosage is 25 mg a day.
For rosacea: Dosages of 50 mg a day are recommended.
For migraines: Even higher amounts may be needed—up to 400 mg a day.

Many one-a-day vitamins meet the RDA for riboflavin; high-potency multivitamins may contain much higher amounts—30 mg or more. Mixed vitamin B formulas typically contain 50 or 100 mg of riboflavin along with other B vitamins, including niacin, thiamin, vitamins B_6 and B_{12}, and folic acid.

GUIDELINES FOR USE

• Don't take riboflavin with alcohol, which reduces its absorption in the digestive tract.

▼ OTHER SOURCES

Good sources of riboflavin include milk, cheese, yogurt, liver, beef, fish, fortified breads and cereals, avocados, mushrooms, and eggs.

FACTS & TIPS

■ Americans get about half their riboflavin from milk and other dairy products.

■ Milk stored in a clear glass bottle loses three-fourths of its riboflavin after just a few hours because the vitamin is extremely sensitive to light. That's one reason why milk comes in opaque bottles or cardboard cartons.

■ Eating a well-balanced diet is especially important for elderly people because many of them are deficient in riboflavin.

LATEST FINDINGS

■ In a recent European study, 55 patients who suffered two to eight migraines per month were given 400 mg of riboflavin a day. After three months, patients experienced, on average, 37% fewer headaches—a rate commonly achieved only with prescription migraine drugs. But riboflavin has far fewer side effects than those drugs, and at around 50 or 60 cents for a daily 400 mg dose, it's much cheaper.

DID YOU KNOW?

You'd have to drink approximately 72 eight-ounce glasses of milk to get 30 mg of riboflavin, the amount found in many high-potency multivitamins.

SAW PALMETTO *(Serenoa repens)*

Native Americans regularly consumed this herb as a food and used it as a tonic, so they were probably not plagued by prostate problems. Long a favorite in Europe, saw palmetto is now one of the ten best-selling supplements in the United States as well. This is definitely an herb with a man's troubles in mind.

COMMON USES

■ Eases frequent nighttime urination, weak urine flow, and other symptoms of an enlarged prostate.

■ Relieves prostate inflammation.

■ May boost immunity and treat urinary tract infections.

FORMS

■ Capsule

■ Tablet

■ Softgel

■ Liquid

■ Dried herb/Tea

▼ WHAT IT IS

The saw palmetto, a small palm tree that grows wild from Texas to South Carolina, gets its name from the spiny saw-toothed stems that lie at the base of each leaf. With a life span of nearly 700 years, the plant seems almost indestructible, resisting drought, insect infestation, and fire.

Its medicinal properties are derived from the blue-black berries, which are usually harvested in August and September. This process is sometimes hazardous: Harvesters can easily be cut by the razor-sharp leaf stems, and they risk being bitten by the diamondback rattlesnakes that make their home in the shade of this scrubby palm.

▼ WHAT IT DOES

Saw palmetto has a long history of folk use. Native Americans valued it for treating disorders of the urinary tract. Early colonists, noting the vitality of animals who fed on the berries, gave the fruits to frail individuals as a general tonic. Through the years, it's also been employed to relieve persistent coughs and improve digestion. Today, saw palmetto's main claim to fame rests on its ability to relieve the symptoms of an enlarged prostate gland—a use verified by a number of reputable scientific studies.

MAJOR BENEFITS

In Italy, Germany, France, and other countries, doctors routinely prescribe saw palmetto for the benign (non-cancerous) enlargement of the prostate gland known medically as BPH, which stands for "benign prostatic hyperplasia," or "hypertrophy."

When the walnut-size prostate gland becomes enlarged, a common condition that affects more than half of men over age 50, it can press on the urethra, the tube that carries urine from the bladder through the prostate and out the penis. The resulting symptoms typically include frequent

ALERT

SIDE EFFECTS

• Although relatively uncommon, possible side effects include mild abdominal pain, nausea, dizziness, and headache.

• In men, reduced sex drive and impotence may occur, but are less likely than with prescription drugs for BPH (benign prostatic hyperplasia).

• Very rarely, men develop breast enlargement. If side effects occur, lower the dose or stop taking the herb altogether.

CAUTION

• Anyone finding blood in the urine or having trouble urinating should see a doctor before taking saw palmetto. These symptoms could be related to prostate cancer.

• Because saw palmetto affects hormone levels, men with prostate cancer or anyone taking hormones should discuss use of the herb with a doctor.

• Women who are pregnant and breast-feeding should not take the herb.

• **Reminder:** If you have a medical condition, talk to your doctor before taking supplements.

urination (especially at night), weak urine flow, painful urination, and difficulty emptying the bladder completely. Researchers believe that saw palmetto relieves the symptoms of BPH in various ways. Most importantly, it appears to alter levels of various hormones that cause prostate cells to multiply. In addition, the herb may act to curb inflammation and reduce tissue swelling.

Studies have found that saw palmetto produces fewer side effects (such as impotence) and quicker results than the conventional prostate drug finasteride (Proscar). Saw palmetto took only about 30 days to become effective, compared with at least six months for the prescription medication.

ADDITIONAL BENEFITS
Although there is strong evidence that saw palmetto relieves the symptoms of BPH, other potential benefits of this herb are more speculative. Saw palmetto has been used to treat certain inflammations of the prostate (prostatitis). In the lab, this herb boosts the immune system's ability to kill bacteria, which suggests that it may be a potential treatment for prostate or urinary tract infections.

Because saw palmetto affects levels of cancer-promoting hormones, scientists are also investigating its possible role in preventing prostate cancer.

▼ HOW TO TAKE IT

DOSAGE
The usual dosage is 160 mg standardized extract twice a day in pill or capsule form or 1 teaspoon liquid extract twice a day.

Be careful if you're thinking about taking higher amounts: Scientific studies have not examined the effects of daily doses above 320 mg.

Choose saw palmetto supplements made from extracts standardized to contain 85% to 95% fatty acids and sterols—the active ingredients in the berries that are responsible for the herb's therapeutic effects.

GUIDELINES FOR USE
• Because saw palmetto has a bitter taste, those using the liquid form may want to dilute the extract in a small amount of water.

• The herb can be taken with or without food, although taking it with breakfast or dinner will minimize the risk of stomach upset.

• Although some herbal healers recommend sipping a tea made from saw palmetto, such a brew may not contain therapeutic amounts of the active ingredients—and so it will provide few real benefits for the treatment of BPH.

SHOPPING HINTS
■ Read the label carefully when buying a "Men's Formula." Although most contain saw palmetto, they usually also include a number of other herbs or nutrients, and some of these may not be right for you. In addition, the amount of saw palmetto in these products may be too small to be of any use.

LATEST FINDINGS
■ In an international study of 1,000 men with moderate BPH, two-thirds benefited from taking either a prescription prostate drug (Proscar) or saw palmetto for six months. Those using the herb had fewer problems with side effects associated with the drug, such as reduced libido and impotence. However, the conventional medication significantly reduced the size of the prostate, whereas the effect of saw palmetto was much less dramatic, particularly in men who had very large prostates. The study authors concluded that the herb may be most appropriate when the gland is only slightly or moderately enlarged.

DID YOU KNOW?
The cost of daily doses of saw palmetto is one-third to one-half that of conventional prostate drugs.

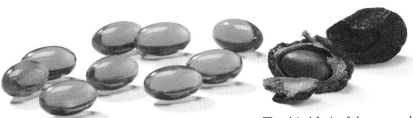

The dried fruit of the saw palmetto tree, often processed into softgels, provides a potent remedy for prostate complaints.

SELENIUM

Although researchers didn't discover the importance of this trace mineral until 1979, selenium quickly gained prominence as a potentially powerful cancer fighter. Today many experts believe selenium to be such a potent antioxidant that it could prove to be a key disease-fighting nutrient for a host of other ailments as well.

COMMON USES

■ Helps in the prevention of cancer and heart disease.

■ Protects against cataracts and macular degeneration.

■ Fights viral infections; reduces the severity of cold sores and shingles; may slow the progression of HIV/AIDS.

■ Helps relieve rheumatoid arthritis and lupus symptoms.

FORMS

■ Capsule
■ Tablet

▼ WHAT IT IS

A trace mineral essential for many body processes, selenium is found in soil. In the body, selenium is present in virtually every cell but is most abundant in the kidneys, liver, spleen, pancreas, and testes.

▼ WHAT IT DOES

Selenium acts as an antioxidant, blocking the rogue molecules known as free radicals that damage DNA. It's part of an antioxidant enzyme (called glutathione peroxidase) that protects cells against environmental and dietary toxins, and is often included in antioxidant "cocktails" with vitamins C and E. This combination may help guard against a wide range of disorders—from cancer, heart disease, cataracts, and macular degeneration to strokes and even aging—thought to be caused by free-radical damage.

MAJOR BENEFITS

Selenium has received a lot of attention recently for its role in combating cancer. A dramatic five-year study conducted at Cornell University and the University of Arizona showed that 200 mcg of selenium daily resulted in 63% fewer prostate tumors, 58% fewer colorectal cancers, 46% fewer lung malignancies, and a 39% overall decrease in cancer deaths. In other studies, selenium showed promise in preventing cancers of the ovaries, cervix, rectum, bladder, esophagus, pancreas, and liver, as well as against leukemia.

Studies of cancer patients indicate that people with the lowest selenium levels developed more tumors, had a higher rate of disease recurrence, a greater risk of cancer spreading, and a shorter overall survival rate than those with high blood levels of selenium.

Additionally, selenium can protect the heart, primarily by reducing the "stickiness" of the blood and decreasing the risk of clotting—which, in turn, lowers the risk of heart attack and stroke. Also, selenium increases the ratio of HDL ("good") cholesterol to LDL ("bad") cholesterol, critical for a healthy heart.

Smokers or those who've already had a heart attack or stroke may gain the greatest cardiovascular benefits from selenium supplements, though everyone can profit from taking selenium in a daily high-potency multivitamin.

ALERT

CAUTION

• Don't exceed recommended doses: In some people, taking selenium long term—at doses of 900 mcg a day—can cause serious side effects, such as skin rashes, nausea, fatigue, hair loss, fingernail abnormalities, and depression.

• **Reminder:** If you have a medical condition, talk to your doctor before taking supplements.

ADDITIONAL BENEFITS

Selenium may be useful in preventing cataracts and macular degeneration, the leading causes of impaired vision or blindness in older Americans. It is also vital for converting thyroid hormone, which is needed for the proper functioning of every cell in the body, from a less active form (called T4) to its active form (known as T3).

In addition, selenium is essential for a healthy immune system, assisting the body in defending itself against harmful bacteria and viruses, as well as cancer cells. Its immune-boosting effects may play a role in fighting the herpes viruses that are responsible for cold sores and shingles, and it is also being studied for possible effectiveness against HIV, the virus that causes AIDS.

When combined with vitamin E, selenium appears to have some anti-inflammatory benefits as well. These two nutrients may improve chronic conditions such as rheumatoid arthritis, psoriasis, lupus, and eczema.

▼ HOW MUCH YOU NEED

The RDA for selenium is 55 mcg for men and women daily. To produce major benefits, up to 600 mcg a day may be needed.

IF YOU GET TOO LITTLE

Most Americans consume enough selenium in their daily diet, so deficiencies of this mineral are rare. Falling below the RDA, however, may lead to higher incidences of cancer, heart disease, immune problems, and inflammatory conditions of all kinds, particularly those affecting the skin. Insufficient amounts of selenium during pregnancy could increase the risk of birth defects (especially those involving the heart) or, possibly, sudden infant death syndrome (SIDS). Early symptoms of selenium deficiency include muscular weakness and fatigue.

IF YOU GET TOO MUCH

It's hard to get too much selenium from your diet, but if you're taking this mineral in supplement form, remember that the margin of safety between a therapeutic dose of selenium (up to 600 mcg a day) and a toxic dose (as little as 900 mcg) is quite small compared with other nutrients. Specific symptoms of selenium toxicity include nervousness, depression, nausea and vomiting, a garlicky odor to the breath and perspiration, and a loss of hair and fingernails.

▼ HOW TO TAKE IT

DOSAGE

Most experts agree the optimum dose for long-term use of selenium should fall between 100 mcg and 400 mcg daily. Up to 600 mcg daily may be taken for a limited time as a treatment for viral infections or as part of a cancer treatment program.

GUIDELINES FOR USE

• Vitamin E greatly enhances selenium's effectiveness; be sure that you get 400 IU of it daily.

▼ OTHER SOURCES

The most abundant sources of selenium include Brazil nuts, seafood, poultry, and meats. Grains, particularly oats and brown rice, may also have significant amounts of the mineral, depending on the selenium content of the soil in which they were grown.

SHOPPING HINTS

■ If you're taking selenium for its antioxidant benefits, consider trying an antioxidant blend formula. These contain selenium along with other potent antioxidants, such as alpha-lipoic acid, coenzyme Q_{10}, NAC (N-acetylcysteine), grape seed and green tea extracts, vitamins C and E, and beta-carotene.

LATEST FINDINGS

■ Recent studies show that in the test tube selenium works relatively quickly, helping cells grow and die at normal rates and protecting them from becoming cancerous. Experts suspect that selenium's cancer-fighting benefits may be fairly fast-acting in the body as well.

■ According to the journal *Agriculture Research*, studies in mice show that a deficiency in either of the antioxidants selenium or vitamin E can convert a latent, inactive virus into its active, disease-causing form. This may explain why selenium is effective against cold sores and shingles, which are both caused by reactivation of a dormant herpes virus.

DID YOU KNOW?

A single Brazil nut contains a whopping 120 mcg of selenium, which is at least 10 times more by weight than is present in any other food, and about twice the RDA for this mineral. Four ounces of red snapper, another good source of selenium, supplies 200 mcg.

SHARK CARTILAGE

Not usually friends to humans, sharks are finally getting a warmer welcome, largely thanks to a tough, rubbery material in their skeletons. Though myriad claims are made for shark cartilage—most spectacularly that it cures cancer—its actual role in the treatment of disease remains uncertain.

COMMON USES
 May help fight cancer.

■ May ease arthritic joint pain, temper the skin lesions of psoriasis, and help heal cold sores.

FORMS
■ Tablet
■ Capsule
■ Powder

▼ WHAT IT IS

Bone forms the framework of the human body. Cartilage does the same for sharks. This elastic substance, which is softer than bone but tough and fibrous, is found in people as well: in the nose, for example, and around the joints. In recent years, shark cartilage products have become popular worldwide as a much-hyped remedy for a variety of ills. Harvested from the head and fins, the cartilage is cleaned, dried, and ground into a fine white powder.

There is much debate, however, about whether the supplement is effective. Solid evidence proving its health benefits lags significantly behind the glowing testimonials. What's more, ecological concern is mounting because shark populations around the globe appear to be declining rapidly due to overfishing.

▼ WHAT IT DOES

Most researchers greet the claims made for shark cartilage—from curing cancer and AIDS to healing arthritis and herpes—with skepticism. Some believe that stomach acids digest shark cartilage, rendering oral supplements ineffective; others say that even if the body does absorb the cartilage, it has no demonstrable therapeutic benefits.

If shark cartilage does contain healing ingredients, they are present, at best, only in very small amounts. Though a few promising studies have been conducted, additional research is needed to confirm—or disprove—the effectiveness of this controversial supplement.

MAJOR BENEFITS
Research dating back to the 1980s sparked interest in this supplement's greatest claim to fame: its supposed ability to battle cancer. Observing that sharks rarely get cancer, investigators began studying various substances from sharks. In their research they noted that shark cartilage blocks the growth of new blood vessels.

Because blood-vessel growth is essential for tumors—providing them with an oxygen-rich blood supply that allows them to survive and grow—the researchers speculated that the cartilage might fight cancer. (Cancer therapies that inhibit blood vessel growth recently became headline news when

ALERT

SIDE EFFECTS
• Even when taken in large amounts, shark cartilage does not seem to produce any toxic reactions.

CAUTION
• Because it may interfere with new blood vessel growth, shark cartilage should not be used by women who are pregnant or breast-feeding; by anyone who has suffered a heart attack or stroke; or by those who have had recent surgery.

• **Reminder:** If you have a medical condition, talk to your doctor before taking supplements.

two drugs that shrink tumors—called angiostatin and endostatin—were isolated in the laboratory.)

Other theories have been advanced for shark cartilage's supposed anticancer effects, and studies in test tubes and animals suggest that it may have some cancer-fighting benefits. But what works in the test tube or in animals is often a far cry from what works in people: Studies have generally failed to show any significant benefits to people with cancer, even when shark cartilage was given in very high doses. In fact, a leading maker of shark cartilage supplements recently admitted that the substance is "probably not effective" for cancer.

ADDITIONAL BENEFITS

Shark cartilage may also have anti-inflammatory properties that make it useful for treating diseases such as rheumatoid arthritis and the skin ailment psoriasis. In one study, animals given a shark cartilage extract experienced less pain and inflammation from substances that irritate the skin.

Shark cartilage may also ease symptoms of osteoarthritis by facilitating the delivery of cartilage-building nutrients to the joints, thereby stimulating cartilage repair while reducing cartilage breakdown. (Most doctors, however, believe there are more effective remedies for this purpose, such as the nutritional supplement glucosamine.)

Due to its possible immune-boosting effects, the supplement has also been proposed as a treatment for cold sores and other herpes infections.

▼ HOW TO TAKE IT

DOSAGE

For disorders such as arthritis: Dosages of about 2,000 mg of shark cartilage three times a day are sometimes recommended.
For cancer: Practitioners sometimes recommend doses as high as 1,000 mg per 2.2 pounds of body weight, which would mean 68,000 mg for someone weighing 150 pounds—a substantial expense for a supplement with unproven value.

GUIDELINES FOR USE

• Some researchers suggest taking the supplement on an empty stomach to minimize exposure to stomach acids that could destroy active ingredients in the shark cartilage.

• Because of the large amounts recommended to treat cancer (in some cases the equivalent of more than 100 capsules a day), the powder form may be more convenient and inexpensive.

• Those concerned about the fishy taste of many products may find tablets or capsules the best options.

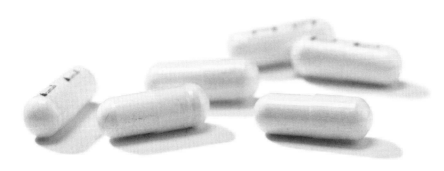

SHOPPING HINTS

■ Many shark cartilage products contain few active ingredients because they are extensively diluted with binding agents and fillers. Read the label carefully to see what you're getting.

LATEST FINDINGS

■ According to a recent Canadian study, shark cartilage helps to treat psoriasis, a condition that's marked by excessive inflammation and growth of new blood vessels in the skin. To mimic the disease, investigators applied a chemical irritant to the arms of nine healthy volunteers. When spread on the skin prior to the application of the irritant, an extract of shark cartilage effectively curtailed inflammation. In a follow-up study, the extract also soothed the rashes of those who actually had psoriasis.

■ Although shark cartilage is often promoted for its cancer-fighting properties, the supplement appeared to have no effect in a study conducted by the Cancer Treatment Research Foundation. Some 60 patients with breast, colon, lung, prostate, and other advanced cancers took numerous spoonfuls of shark cartilage three times a day. Over 10 months, the supplement had no discernible effect on their tumors.

DID YOU KNOW?

In Japan, shark fin soup is thought to be a longevity booster.

SIBERIAN GINSENG (*Eleutherococcus senticosus*)

This ancient Chinese tonic, rediscovered by the Russians after World War II, helps an individual withstand stress more effectively. A series of recent studies have shown that this herb appears to benefit the whole body, sharpening physical and mental performance and restoring vitality during times of overwork or illness.

COMMON USES

- Combats stress-related illness.
- Fights fatigue; restores energy.
- Enhances immunity and helps relieve symptoms of chronic fatigue syndrome and fibromyalgia.
- Supports sexual function; may improve fertility in both sexes.
- Eases symptoms of menopause.
- May boost mental alertness in people with Alzheimer's disease.

FORMS

- Tablet
- Capsule
- Softgel
- Tincture/Liquid
- Powder
- Dried herb/Tea

WHAT IT IS

Also called eleuthero, Siberian ginseng is a distant botanical cousin of Panax ginseng, which is the better known of the two. Although not as revered (or expensive) as the Panax species, Siberian ginseng has been used in China for thousands of years to enhance the body's vital energy (*qi*), restore memory, and prevent colds and flu. It is derived from *Eleutherococcus senticosus*, a plant native to eastern Russia, China, Korea, and Japan; supplements are usually made from the dried roots.

Siberian ginseng gained prominence among Western doctors in the 1950s, after a Russian health researcher, I. I. Brekhman, completed experiments examining its effects on thousands of men and women. His studies demonstrated that Siberian ginseng could help healthy people withstand physical stress, improve their immune systems, and increase their mental and physical performance. Subsequent research revealed the herb's potential for treating specific ailments.

WHAT IT DOES

Siberian ginseng contains substances that exert beneficial effects on the adrenals (the small glands on top of the kidneys that secrete stress-fighting hormones). It also raises energy levels and enhances immunity. Studies show that the herb is effective in protecting against all kinds of physical stresses: heat, cold, even radiation. It heightens mental alertness and allows the mind to focus in adverse situations. By reducing the effects of stress and supporting the immune system, Siberian ginseng may also be of value in decreasing the risk of many chronic illnesses.

MAJOR BENEFITS

Siberian ginseng is often recommended as a general revitalizer for people who are fatigued (including those recovering from illness and those who are overworked). It's also suggested for people whose ability to work is impaired, or for those whose concentration is weak.

Studies in Russia involving 2,100 healthy men and women ages 19 to 72 who were given extracts of the herb found that Siberian ginseng improved the

ALERT

SIDE EFFECTS
- The herb appears to be very safe at recommended doses. In rare cases, it may cause mild diarrhea, menstrual irregularities, or agitation.

- Some report feeling restless after taking Siberian ginseng, so don't use it too close to bedtime.

CAUTION
- Siberian ginseng may interfere in hazardous ways with heart medications including digoxin and antihypertensives. Consult your doctor.

- Don't take while menstruating and stop taking it if you become pregnant.

- **Reminder:** If you have a medical condition, talk to your doctor before taking supplements.

following: physical labor performance; accuracy at proofreading; radio telegraphists' speed and precision in noisy surroundings; the ability of humans to adapt to hot temperatures, as well as to a high-altitude, low-oxygen environment; and their ability to withstand the nausea of motion sickness.

Because it also enhances immunity, Siberian ginseng is frequently included in nutritional support programs for people with chronic fatigue syndrome or fibromyalgia. In addition, it may benefit people in the early stages of Alzheimer's disease by increasing mental alertness.

ADDITIONAL BENEFITS
By altering hormone levels and toning the uterus, Siberian ginseng may play a role in treating menstrual irregularities and menopausal symptoms. Taken between menstrual periods, it may also be useful in preventing female infertility.

The herb may be suitable as a fertility aid for men as well. When alternated with Panax ginseng, it may be of value for some cases of impotence.

Traditionally, the Chinese have utilized Siberian ginseng to suppress colds and flu; the herb's efficacy may partly be related to its ability to improve the immune system. Russian studies support this use. In a very large study, more than 13,000 auto workers who took the herb one winter reported suffering 40% fewer respiratory tract infections during that period than in previous winters.

Siberian ginseng has also been employed to treat certain heart conditions and to lower blood sugar; test-tube studies suggest that Siberian ginseng may help protect against some types of cancer or boost the effects of conventional chemotherapy drugs. More studies are needed to verify these and other potential benefits.

▼ HOW TO TAKE IT

DOSAGE
For stress, fatigue, and other complaints: Take 100 to 300 mg of a standardized extract two or three times a day or 1 teaspoon of liquid extract once or twice a day.
For menstrual disorders: Use Siberian ginseng along with herbs such as chasteberry, dong quai, and licorice. Commercial combinations are available.

GUIDELINES FOR USE
• Siberian ginseng can be taken on a long-term basis. However, some authorities suggest using it for three months and then stopping for a week or two.

• German health authorities do not recommend Siberian ginseng for people who have high blood pressure. There are few studies, however, that indicate any adverse reactions within this group.

SHOPPING HINTS
■ Buy standardized Siberian ginseng (eleuthero) extracts from a reputable company so you'll get a quality product. Look for extracts with an eleutheroside content of at least 0.8%.

■ Siberian ginseng is often added to "Adrenal Gland" formulas that are intended to combat stress. Look for the herb in combination with licorice, pantothenic acid, and other ingredients.

■ Avoid high-potency formulas of Siberian ginseng that exceed recommended daily doses. High doses (more than 900 mg a day) can cause insomnia, irritability, nervousness, and anxiety.

LATEST FINDINGS
■ In Germany, Siberian ginseng is approved for use as an invigorating tonic for fatigue, weakness, an inability to work, impaired concentration, and convalescence from illness. But it may not be effective at enabling a fit and well-nourished American athlete to run any faster or longer. When 20 highly trained distance runners were given Siberian ginseng, they didn't perform any better in treadmill tests than their peers on placebos.

DID YOU KNOW?
After the Chernobyl nuclear accident, many Russians were offered Siberian ginseng to help minimize the effects of the radiation.

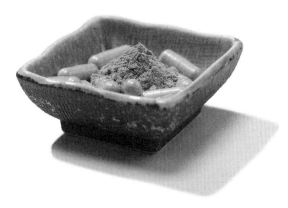

SOY ISOFLAVONES

Soy has shown great promise in reducing the uncomfortable hot flashes associated with menopause. Used as a phytoestrogen in Asia for hundreds of years, it is now the subject of new research indicating that it may also help protect against certain chronic diseases, including osteoporosis, heart disease, and some cancers.

COMMON USES

■ Reduce the frequency and severity of hot flashes and other symptoms related to menopause.

■ May protect against coronary heart disease.

■ May forestall certain cancers.

■ May help prevent osteoporosis.

FORMS

■ Capsule

■ Tablet

■ Soy protein powder

▼ WHAT IT IS

Found in soybean products such as tofu and soy milk, and sold in supplement form, isoflavones are powerful compounds known as phytoestrogens. These plant-based substances are chemically similar to the hormone estrogen (produced in the body), but are much weaker. Phytoestrogens, however, can bind to estrogen receptors in the cells and produce various important health benefits.

Most research on soy isoflavones has been done with people who regularly ate soy products. Therefore, even though most supplements contain the major isoflavones in soybeans (genistein and daidzein), it's not clear whether isoflavones are the only beneficial compounds in soy.

▼ WHAT IT DOES

As phytoestrogens, soy isoflavones have two important effects. First, when estrogen levels are high, phytoestrogens can block the more potent forms of estrogen produced by the body and may help prevent hormone-driven diseases, such as breast cancer. Second, when estrogen levels are low, as they are after menopause, phytoestrogens can substitute for the body's own estrogen, possibly reducing hot flashes and preserving bones. Soy isoflavones may also have antioxidant and anticoagulant effects.

PREVENTION

Research indicates that soybean products help protect against heart disease by lowering LDL ("bad") cholesterol and significantly increasing HDL ("good") cholesterol. Soy seems most effective in people with high cholesterol levels. In those with near-normal cholesterol levels, its effects are less powerful, and larger amounts are needed to produce the same benefits. Soy products may also inhibit the oxidation of LDL cholesterol, the first step in the accumulation of artery-clogging plaque. In addition, laboratory studies

ALERT

SIDE EFFECTS

• Soy products, even in large quantities, are not known to produce side effects other than occasional mild gas.

• The small percentage of people who are allergic to soybeans should avoid all soy supplements and soy-based foods.

CAUTION

• Consult your doctor before taking soy supplements to prevent cancer.

• Pregnant or breast-feeding women should not take soy isoflavone supplements, given the estrogenlike effects of this concentrated form. Soy-rich foods are safe, however.

• The potential health risks of soy isoflavones in concentrated capsule form are unclear. Consult your doctor for guidance, particularly if you have a strong family history of breast cancer; laboratory findings indicate some risk, although more research is needed.

• **Reminder:** If you have a medical condition, talk to your doctor before taking supplements.

show the genistein in soy helps prevent blood clots from forming.

In Asian countries where soy is a dietary staple, rates of certain cancers are much lower than they are in the United States. Preliminary studies indicate that regular consumption of soy foods may protect against cancers of the breast, prostate, and endometrium. And in animal studies, adding soy protein to the diet significantly reduces tumor formation and the likelihood that cancer, once developed, will spread.

The phytoestrogens in the soy are most likely responsible for this effect. Researchers speculate that the isoflavone genistein may block a protein called tyrosine kinase, which promotes the growth and proliferation of tumor cells. This effect may be why soy is also associated with a lower risk of prostate cancer in men. Genistein has potent antioxidant properties as well, and for these reasons, it may one day prove useful against cancer—though more research is clearly needed.

ADDITIONAL BENEFITS

Studies show that hot flashes and other symptoms of menopause are relatively rare in Asia, where women generally eat a lot of soy products. In addition, in one Western study, women who added 45 grams of soy flour to their daily diet experienced a notable 40% reduction in the occurrence of menopause-related hot flashes.

Interestingly, soy isoflavones may also help women maintain bone density. One study of postmenopausal women found that consuming 40 grams of soy protein a day resulted in a significant increase in bone mineral density in the spine, an area often weakened by osteoporosis (brittle-bone disease).

▼ HOW TO TAKE IT

DOSAGE

Experts don't know the amount of soy isoflavones needed to produce a therapeutic effect. In Asian countries, the isoflavone consumption ranges from 25 to 200 mg a day. Some researchers now believe that an intake of 50 to 120 mg a day might be the minimum amount necessary.

The supplements on the market vary in the types of isoflavones they contain and the total amount of isoflavones per pill. Choose a product that supplies a mixture of isoflavones—it should include both genistein and daidzein—and take enough pills to obtain 50 to 100 mg isoflavones a day.

GUIDELINES FOR USE

• Most experts recommend that you try to get your soy isoflavones from soy foods. In addition to their isoflavone content, these foods are good sources of protein, so they can replace red meat and other foods high in saturated fat.

• The amount of isoflavones in soybeans—and therefore any product made from them—varies. Eating one to two servings of soy products a day is probably sufficient. (A serving equals: 3½ ounces tofu or miso, 1 cup soy milk, or ½ cup soy flour, cooked soybeans, or texturized vegetable protein.) If eating this much soy is not to your taste, you might want to get your isoflavones from a combination of foods and supplements.

• Another alternative is soy powder, which contains both soy protein and isoflavones; mix it into juice, milk, or shakes. Take soy supplements with a large glass of warm water right before eating breakfast and dinner.

FACTS & TIPS

■ A diet high in fiber may interfere with the absorption of isoflavones. If you eat a high-fiber diet, be sure to increase your consumption of soy supplements or soy foods.

■ Even though they're made from soybeans, soy sauce and soybean oil contain no isoflavones.

LATEST FINDINGS

■ In a recent study, people with moderately high cholesterol levels drank a daily "milkshake" containing 25 grams of soy protein, either with or without isoflavones. After nine weeks, those who consumed the isoflavone-rich shake experienced, on average, a 5% reduction in LDL ("bad") cholesterol levels. People with the highest LDL levels had an 11% drop. (For each 10% to 15% drop in LDL levels, the risk of a heart attack decreases 20% to 25%.)

■ Women who ate the most soy products and other foods rich in phytoestrogens reduced their risk of endometrial cancer by 54%, according to one study. Soy products may be especially important for those women who have never been pregnant.

SPIRULINA AND KELP

Health enthusiasts are looking to the lakes and seas for algae and plant proteins that are powerful food supplements. Although spirulina and kelp have inspired hype as well as hope, these aquatic plants actually do contain various helpful substances, with benefits ranging from sweetening the breath to helping the thyroid.

COMMON USES

Spirulina
- Treats bad breath.
- Adds protein, vitamins, and minerals to the diet.

Kelp
- Treats underactive thyroid.
- Provides essential nutrients.

FORMS
- Capsule
- Tablet
- Powder
- Tincture
- Liquid

▼ WHAT IT IS

Spirulina and kelp are two very different types of aquatic algae. The smaller of the two, spirulina (also known as blue-green algae), is actually a single-celled microorganism, or microalga, that closely resembles a bacterium. Because its spiral-shaped filaments are rich in the plant pigment chlorophyll, spirulina turns the lakes and ponds where it grows a dark blue-green.

Kelp is another beneficial protector—one that comes from the sea. Derived from various species of brown algae known as *Fucus* or *Laminaria*, this long-stemmed seaweed is a prime source of iodine, crucial in preventing thyroid problems.

▼ WHAT IT DOES

Spirulina and kelp have been used medicinally for thousands of years in China. Their devotees make many claims—ranging from increased libido to reduced hair loss—but most of these benefits remain highly speculative. The algae do, however, have some confirmed powers.

MAJOR BENEFITS
Because it is a prime source of chlorophyll, spirulina is ideal for combating one of life's most bothersome complaints: bad breath. It can be an extremely effective remedy, provided the condition is not due to gum disease or chronic sinusitis. Many commercial chlorophyll breath fresheners contain spirulina as a key ingredient.

The high iodine content of kelp makes it useful for treating an underactive thyroid that's caused by a shortage of iodine. This remedy is rarely necessary, however, because iodized salt supplies plenty of this mineral.

Kelp is also marketed as a weight-loss aid, but it's probably effective only in the really rare cases when weight gain is secondary to an iodine-deficient, underactive thyroid. Kelp should be taken only under the close supervision of a physician for the treatment of thyroid disorders.

ALERT

SIDE EFFECTS
- Occasionally, nausea or diarrhea develops in those taking spirulina or kelp; if this side effect occurs, lower the dose or stop using the algae.

- Up to 3% of the population is sensitive to iodine and may experience adverse reactions to long-term ingestion of kelp—including a painful enlargement of the thyroid gland that disappears once kelp consumption is discontinued.

CAUTION
- Kelp may aggravate the condition of people taking medication for an overactive thyroid. Consult your doctor before taking this supplement with any thyroid medication.

- **Reminder:** If you have a medical condition, talk to your doctor before taking supplements.

ADDITIONAL BENEFITS

Sometimes spirulina and kelp are included in vegetarian and macrobiotic diets. Spirulina contains protein, vitamins (including B$_{12}$ and folic acid), carotenoids, and other nutrients. In addition to iodine, kelp provides carotenoids, as well as fatty acids, potassium, magnesium, calcium, iron, and other nutrients. However, the concentrations of all these substances appear to be fairly low. There are many less expensive—and better tasting—sources of vitamins and minerals than spirulina and kelp, including an array of common garden vegetables.

Various other claims are made for kelp and spirulina—that they boost energy, relieve arthritis, enhance liver function, prevent heart disease and certain types of cancer, boost immunity, suppress HIV and AIDS, and protect cells against damage from X rays or heavy metals, But most studies on these supplements have been done in test tubes or with animals, and more research is needed.

▼ HOW TO TAKE IT

DOSAGE

As a concentrated nutritional source: Use a commercial, chlorophyll-rich "green" drink (the label will often say if the chlorophyll is derived in part from spirulina) and follow package directions regarding preparation.

To freshen the breath with spirulina: Mix a teaspoon of spirulina powder in half a glass of water. Swish the liquid around the mouth, then swallow it. Alternatively, chew a tablet thoroughly, then ingest it. Repeat three or four times a day, or as needed.

To use kelp for an underactive thyroid: Use only when recommended by your doctor; if iodine is needed, your doctor can prescribe an appropriate dose. Powder forms dissolve easily in water, though some people don't like the taste. Tablets, capsules, and tinctures are equally effective.

GUIDELINES FOR USE

• Take with food to minimize the chances of digestive upset.

• Pregnant or breast-feeding women may want to avoid kelp because of its high iodine content, though spirulina seems to be very safe.

SHOPPING HINTS

■ Look for commercial breath fresheners that contain spirulina as one of the first listed ingredients. Its rich chlorophyll content is a safe and effective natural way to freshen your breath.

■ Always check the expiration date on a package of kelp, because the iodine content may decline with storage. In one test, no iodine could be detected in kelp tablets that had been on a shelf for a year and a half.

FACTS & TIPS

■ Don't harvest your own spirulina or kelp from the wild. Coastal or aquatic colonies of the algae may be contaminated with industrial waste or sewage and contain concentrated levels of lead, mercury, cadmium, or other dangerous toxins.

DID YOU KNOW?

Kelp cultivated for supplements in the United States is commonly called "rockweed." It is olive green to brown in color and generally grows three to six feet long—much smaller than the more common "kelp" frequently seen along U.S. coastlines.

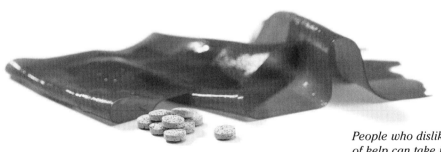

People who dislike the taste of kelp can take it in pill form.

ST. JOHN'S WORT *(Hypericum perforatum)*

Ancient Greeks and Romans believed that this herb could deter evil spirits. Today, St. John's wort has found new and widespread popularity as a natural antidepressant, a gentle alternative to conventional medications with far fewer side effects. Experts believe this herb works by boosting levels of a key brain chemical called

COMMON USES

- Treats depression.
- Helps fight off infections.
- May help treat premenstrual syndrome (PMS) and fibromyalgia.
- Helps relieve chronic pain.
- Soothes hemorrhoids.
- May aid in weight loss.

FORMS

- Tablet
- Capsule
- Softgel
- Liquid
- Cream/Ointment

▼ WHAT IT IS

A shrubby perennial bearing bright yellow flowers, St. John's wort is cultivated worldwide. It was named for Saint John the Baptist because it blooms around June 24, the day celebrated as his birthday; "wort" is an old English word for plant.

For centuries, St. John's wort was used to soothe jangled nerves and to help the healing of wounds, burns, and snakebites. Herbal supplements are made from the plant's dried flowers, which contain a number of therapeutic substances, including a healing pigment called hypericin.

▼ WHAT IT DOES

St. John's wort is most often used to treat mild depression. Scientists aren't sure exactly how the herb works, though it's believed to boost levels of the brain chemical serotonin, which is key to mood and emotions.

MAJOR BENEFITS

Several years ago, a careful analysis of 23 different studies of St. John's wort concluded that the herb was as effective as antidepressant drugs—and more effective than a placebo—in the treatment of mild to moderate depression. A recent study, however, showed that St. John's wort was not effective for treating major serious clinical depression. In such cases, conventional antidepressant therapy is appropriate.

St. John's wort may be helpful for many conditions associated with depression too, such as anxiety, stress, premenstrual syndrome (PMS), fibromyalgia, chronic fatigue syndrome, or chronic pain; it may even have some direct pain-relieving effects.

This herb promotes sound sleep and may be especially valuable when depression is marked by fatigue, sleepiness, and low energy levels. It may also aid in treating "wintertime blues" (seasonal affective disorder), a type of depression that develops in the fall and winter and dissipates in the bright sunlight of spring and summer.

 ALERT

SIDE EFFECTS
- While uncommon, side effects can include constipation, upset stomach, fatigue, dry mouth, and dizziness.

- Avoid prolonged exposure to sunlight while taking St. John's wort; it may increase sensitivity to the sun, especially with high doses or prolonged use.

CAUTION
- If you're taking conventional antidepressant drugs, consult your doctor before switching to St. John's wort. Never alter a drug dose on your own.

- A number of prescription and over-the-counter drugs, including various cardiac, transplant, and HIV medications, interact negatively with St. John's wort; always check with your doctor before combining it with any drug.

- If you develop hives or have difficulty breathing (rarely, people have allergic reactions), get immediate medical help.

- **Reminder:** If you have a medical or psychiatric condition, talk to your doctor before taking supplements.

Some people are leery of conventional antidepressants because of their potential for causing undesirable side effects, especially reduced sexual function. St. John's wort has fewer bothersome side effects than these drugs.

St, John's wort seems so promising that the National Institutes of Health (NIH) is now conducting a major study of its effectiveness that involves more than 330 patients who are suffering from depression.

ADDITIONAL BENEFITS

St. John's wort fights bacteria and viruses as well. Research indicates that it may play a key part in combating herpes simplex, influenza, and Epstein-Barr virus (the cause of mononucleosis), and preliminary laboratory studies reveal a possible role for the herb in the fight against AIDS. When an ointment made from St. John's wort is applied to hemorrhoids, it relieves burning and itching. Taken along with the herb ephedra, St. John's wort may also be useful as a weight-loss aid.

▼ HOW TO TAKE IT

DOSAGE

The recommended dose is 300 mg of an extract standardized to contain 0.3% hypericin, three times a day.

In softgels, capsules, or tablets, St. John's wort can be very effective for mild depression.

Supplements containing 450 mg are also available and can be taken twice a day. Opt for standardized extracts whenever possible; they tend to be of higher quality than nonstandardized formulations.

GUIDELINES FOR USE

• Take St. John's wort with food in order to prevent the fairly common side effect of mild stomach irritation.

• In the past, those using the herb were advised not to eat certain foods, including aged cheese and red wine—the same foods best avoided by those taking MAO inhibitors (a type of antidepressant). But recent studies suggest that these foods do not present a problem for those on St. John's wort.

• Like a prescription antidepressant, the herb must build up in your blood before it becomes effective, so be sure to allow at least four weeks to determine whether it works for you. It can be used long term, as needed.

• Though no adverse effects have been reported in pregnant or breast-feeding women using the herb, there have been few studies in this group of patients, so caution is advised.

FACTS & TIPS

■ You can buy a 30-day supply of St. John's wort for under $10—less than a quarter of the cost of popular antidepressant drugs. Choose preparations standardized to contain 0.3% hypericin, the therapeutic ingredient found in the herb.

■ In Germany, where doctors prescribe herbal remedies routinely, St. John's wort is the most common form of antidepressant—and much more popular than conventional antidepressants.

LATEST FINDINGS

■ In a recent study, 50 participants with mild depression were given either St. John's wort or a placebo. After eight weeks, 70% of those on St. John's wort showed marked improvement, versus 45% of those receiving a placebo. No adverse reactions to the herb were noted.

■ Although used for mild and moderate depression, St. John's wort may one day prove effective for more severe cases. A study of 209 people with serious depression found the herb as effective as conventional antidepressants. But more research is needed before the supplement can be recommended for this purpose.

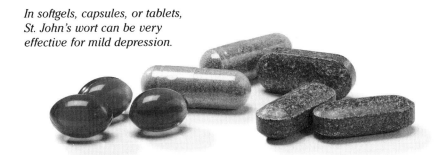

TEA TREE OIL *(Melaleuca alternifolia)*

For centuries, Australian aborigines relied on the leaves of a native tree to fight infections. Dubbed the "tea tree" by English explorer Captain Cook, its leaves produce an oil that is valued throughout the world as a potent antiseptic. Studies have also confirmed its powerful ability to combat bacteria and fungal infections.

COMMON USES

■ Disinfects and promotes the healing of cuts and scrapes.

■ Minimizes scarring.

■ Speeds recovery from bug or spider bites and stings, including bee stings.

■ Fights athlete's foot, fungal nail infections, and yeast infections.

FORMS

■ Oil

■ Gel

■ Cream

■ Vaginal suppository

▼ WHAT IT IS

A champion infection fighter, tea tree oil has a pleasant nutmeglike scent. The oil comes from the leaves of the *Melaleuca alternifolia*, or tea tree, a species that grows only in Australia (and is completely different from the *Camellia* species used to make black, oolong, and green drinking teas).

Extracted through a steam-distillation process, quality tea tree oil contains at least 40% terpinen-4-ol (the active ingredient that is responsible for its healing effects) and less than 5% cineole, a substance that is believed to counteract the medicinal properties of the oil. With the rise of antibiotics after World War II, tea tree oil fell out of favor. Recently, interest in it has revived, and today more than 700 tons of tea tree oil are produced annually.

▼ WHAT IT DOES

Tea tree oil is used topically to treat a variety of common infections. Once applied to the skin, the oil makes it impossible for many disease-causing fungi to survive. Several studies have shown that it fights various bacteria as well, including some that are resistant to powerful antibiotics. Experts think one reason tea tree oil is so effective is that it readily mixes with skin oils, allowing it to attack the infective agent quickly and actively.

MAJOR BENEFITS

Tea tree oil's antiseptic properties are especially useful for treating cuts and scrapes, as well as insect bites and stings. The oil promotes healing of minor wounds, helps prevent infection, and minimizes any future scarring.

As an antifungal agent, tea tree oil fights the fungus *Trichophyton*, the culprit in athlete's foot, jock itch, and some nail infections. It may also be effective against *Candida albicans* and *Trichomonas vaginalis,* two of the organisms that cause vaginal infections. Unfortunately, some fungal infections can be stubborn to treat; in these cases, your doctor may have to prescribe a more potent conventional antifungal medication.

 ALERT

SIDE EFFECTS
• Although tea tree oil can irritate sensitive skin, it otherwise appears to be safe for topical use. Like many herbal oils in pure, undiluted form, it can irritate the eyes and mucous membranes.

CAUTION
• Tea tree oil is for topical use only, and should be kept away from eyes.

• If you accidentally ingest the oil, call a doctor or poison control center immediately.

• Consult your doctor before applying to deep, open wounds.

• **Reminder:** If you have a medical condition, talk to your doctor before using supplements.

ADDITIONAL BENEFITS

Tea tree oil may be beneficial in the treatment of acne. In one study, a gel containing 5% tea tree oil was shown to be as effective against acne as a lotion with 5% benzoyl peroxide, the active ingredient in most over-the-counter acne medications. But there were fewer side effects with tea tree oil: Specifically, it caused less scaling, dryness, and itching than the benzoyl peroxide formula.

Another study found that a solution containing 0.5% tea tree oil offered protection against *Pityrosporum ovale*, a common dandruff-causing fungus. Sometimes tea tree oil is suggested as a treatment for warts, which are caused by viruses, though studies have not confirmed this use.

▼ HOW TO TAKE IT

DOSAGE
To treat athlete's foot, skin wounds, or nail infections: Apply a drop or two of pure, undiluted tea tree oil to the affected areas of the skin or nails two or three times a day. Tea tree oil creams and lotions can also be used for the same purpose.
To treat vaginal yeast infections: Insert a commercially available tea tree oil vaginal suppository every 12 hours, for up to five days. If symptoms of the yeast infection persist, be sure to contact your doctor.

GUIDELINES FOR USE
• Tea tree oil is for topical use only. Never take tea tree oil orally. If you or a child ingests it, call your doctor or a poison control center right away.

• Rarely, tea tree oil can cause an allergic skin rash in some people. Before using the oil for the first time, be sure to dab a small amount onto your inner arm with a cotton swab. If you are allergic, your arm will quickly become red or inflamed. If this response occurs, dilute the tea tree oil by adding a few drops to a tablespoon of bland oil, such as vegetable oil or almond oil, and try the arm test again. If you have no skin reaction, it's safe to apply the diluted tea tree oil elsewhere on the body.

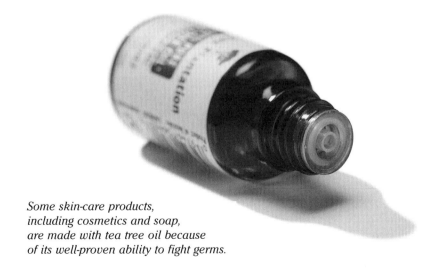

Some skin-care products, including cosmetics and soap, are made with tea tree oil because of its well-proven ability to fight germs.

SHOPPING HINTS

■ A number of shampoos, soaps, and other skin-care products contain tea tree oil, but many have such a small amount that they have little or no bacteria-fighting effect. Contact the manufacturer to find out if any studies on a product's antibacterial effectiveness have been conducted.

■ There is more than one type of tea tree, so when buying tea tree oil, be sure it's derived from *Melaleuca alternifolia*. Oil from other species tends to be high in cineole content and doesn't have the same medicinal properties.

LATEST FINDINGS

■ In one recent test-tube study, tea tree oil (as well as peppermint, cinnamon leaf, and nutmeg oils) was reported to contain substances that are toxic to head lice. Additional study is needed in people before tea tree oil can be recommended to combat lice, particularly in children, who may be especially sensitive to this oil.

■ Swiss researchers found that a special medical preparation of tea tree oil provides protection against cavity-forming bacteria in the mouth. But never use the pure oil in your mouth; it can be irritating and is dangerous if swallowed. Tea tree toothpastes are probably safe because they have so little oil—but for the same reason, they may have limited bacteria-fighting benefits.

THIAMIN

Concerns about getting enough thiamin disappeared in the 1940s, when a law was passed requiring that the B vitamins removed during the milling of refined grains be added back into commercial bread and cereal products. Although severe thiamin deficiency is a thing of the past, even a moderate deficit has health consequences.

COMMON USES

- Aids energy production.
- Promotes healthy nerves.
- May improve mood.
- Strengthens the heart.
- Soothes heartburn.

FORMS

- Tablet
- Capsule

▼ WHAT IT IS

An often overlooked but key member of the B-complex vitamin family, thiamin is known as vitamin B_1 because it was the first B vitamin discovered. Most people get enough thiamin in their diets to meet their basic needs; however, experts believe some people, especially older adults, are mildly deficient in this nutrient.

Thiamin is available as an individual supplement, but it's best to get it from a B-complex supplement, because it works closely with the other B vitamins.

▼ WHAT IT DOES

Thiamin is essential for converting the carbohydrates in foods into energy. It also plays a role in promoting healthy nerves and may be useful in treating certain types of heart disease.

MAJOR BENEFITS

In people with congestive heart failure (CHF), thiamin can help improve the pumping power of the heart. Thiamin levels in the body are depleted by long-term treatment with diuretic drugs, which are often prescribed for CHF patients to reduce the fluid buildup associated with the disease. In one study, CHF patients who took furosemide (a diuretic) were given either 200 mg a day of thiamin or a placebo. After six weeks, the thiamin group showed a 22% improvement.

By helping to maintain healthy nerves, thiamin may minimize numbness and tingling in the hands and feet. This problem frequently plagues people with diabetes or other diseases that cause nerve damage.

ADDITIONAL BENEFITS

In combination with choline and pantothenic acid (also B vitamins), thiamin can enhance the digestive process and provide relief from heartburn. Some researchers think that a thiamin deficiency is linked to mental illnesses, including depression, and that high-dose thiamin supplementation may be beneficial.

Thiamin may also boost memory in people with Alzheimer's disease—but evidence is far from conclusive. However, the confusion that is common in older adults after surgery may be prevented by additional doses of thiamin in the weeks before an operation. Doctors also use thiamin to treat the psychosis related to alcohol withdrawal.

 ALERT

SIDE EFFECTS

- There are no adverse side effects associated with thiamin.

CAUTION

- **Reminder:** If you have a medical or psychiatric condition, talk to your doctor before taking supplements.

Antiseizure medications interfere with the vitamin's absorption, so people taking them may need extra thiamin; this may also reduce the fuzzy thinking that such drugs can cause.

▼ HOW MUCH YOU NEED

To maintain good health and to prevent a thiamin deficiency, the RDA of 1.2 mg a day for men and 1.1 mg a day for women is sufficient. However, higher doses are recommended for therapeutic use.

IF YOU GET TOO LITTLE
A mild thiamin deficiency may go unnoticed. Its symptoms are irritability, weight loss, depression, and muscle weakness. A severe thiamin deficiency causes beriberi, a disease that leads to mental impairment, the wasting away of muscle, paralysis, nerve damage, and eventually death. Once rampant in many countries, beriberi is rare today. It is seen only in parts of Asia where the diet consists mainly of white rice, which is stripped of thiamin and other nutrients during milling. In the United States, thiamin is added to white bread, cereals, pasta, and white rice.

IF YOU GET TOO MUCH
There are no adverse effects associated with high doses of thiamin, because the body is efficient at eliminating excess amounts through the urine.

▼ HOW TO TAKE IT

DOSAGE
Specific disorders can benefit from supplemental thiamin.

For congestive heart failure: Take 200 mg of thiamin daily.
For numbness and tingling: Take 100 mg of thiamin a day (50 mg as part of a B-complex supplement, 50 mg of extra thiamin).
For depression: Take 50 mg daily as part of a B complex.
For heartburn: Take 500 mg a day in the morning.
For alcoholism: Take 150 mg daily (50 mg as part of a B complex and an extra 100 mg).

GUIDELINES FOR USE
• Thiamin is best absorbed in an acid environment. Try to take it with meals, when stomach acid is produced to digest the food you're eating.

• Divide your dose and have it twice a day, because high doses are readily flushed out of the body through urine.

▼ OTHER SOURCES

Lean pork is probably the best dietary source of thiamin, followed by whole grains, dried beans, and nuts and seeds. Enriched grain products also contain thiamin.

FACTS & TIPS
■ If you drink a lot of coffee or tea (decaffeinated or regular), you may need to increase your intake of thiamin. These beverages can deplete your body's thiamin stores.

LATEST FINDINGS
■ Thiamin supplements may boost mood, according to a recent study of young women who were not deficient in thiamin. More than 100 college-age women took either 50 mg of thiamin a day or a placebo for two months. Tests showed that energy levels, alertness, and mood all improved in the thiamin takers, but not in those receiving the placebo.

■ Older people are often mildly deficient in thiamin. A recent study found that taking just 10 mg a day for three months led to lowered blood pressure, weight loss, better-quality sleep, and increased energy levels in people over age 65. No improvements were seen in those individuals who were given a placebo pill.

DID YOU KNOW?
You'd have to eat about 15 cups of shelled sunflower seeds to get a 50 mg dose of thiamin.

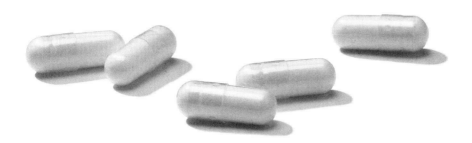

TRACE MINERALS

The old adage that good things come in small packages certainly is true for a group of nutrients known as trace minerals. Though some of these tiny nutritional power-houses are poorly understood, others are known to be essential for everything from strong bones (silicon and boron) to a healthy heart (manganese).

COMMON USES

Boron, silicon, and fluoride

- Aid in building strong bones, teeth, and nails.

Manganese

- Treats heart arrhythmias, osteo-porosis, epileptic seizures, sprains, and back pain.

Vanadium

- May aid people with diabetes.

Molybdenum

- Helps the body use iron.

FORMS

- Tablet
- Capsule
- Powder
- Liquid

▼ WHAT IT IS

Trace minerals are those the body needs in only minuscule amounts. For example, though the average-size person carries around approximately 3 pounds of calcium, the trace mineral manganese weighs in at only 1/2,500 of an ounce.

Some trace minerals, such as copper, iron, magnesium, selenium, and zinc, have been studied extensively and are included elsewhere in this book. Others, discussed here, include boron, fluoride, manganese, molybdenum, silicon, and vanadium.

▼ WHAT IT DOES

The vast majority of trace minerals act as coenzymes, which—in partnership with the proteins known as enzymes—facilitate chemical reactions throughout the body. They aid in forming bones and other tissues, assist in growth and development, make up part of the genetic material DNA, and help the body burn fats and carbohydrates.

PREVENTION

Preliminary evidence suggests that some trace minerals (like their big brother calcium) are good for bones and may be effective against osteo-porosis. Along with silicon, manganese helps build strong bones and connec-tive tissue, the durable substance that holds much of the body together.

Boron may enhance bone health by preventing calcium loss and activating the bone-maintaining hormone estro-gen, whereas vanadium seems to stim-ulate bone-building enzymes. And although fluoride is known mainly for its ability to prevent cavities, some studies suggest that it may also aid in protecting against bone fractures.

ADDITIONAL BENEFITS

In addition to strengthening bones, manganese is part of the enzyme superoxide dismutase, a potent anti-oxidant that plays a role in protecting cells throughout the body. Further-more, some evidence suggests that manganese may benefit people with epilepsy by reducing the likelihood of seizures.

Researchers are investigating the pos-sibility that silicon may be useful in guarding against heart disease. Blood

 ALERT

CAUTION

- Molybdenum may aggravate symptoms of gout.

- Boron can affect hormone levels and should be used with care by those at risk for breast or prostate cancer.

- Manganese may be toxic for anyone with liver or gallbladder disease.

- **Reminder:** If you have a medical condition, talk to your doctor before taking supplements.

vessel walls concentrate this mineral, and people who get more silicon in their diet may have a decreased risk of this disease. Because silicon also strengthens connective tissue, it is sometimes used to nourish hair, skin, and nails. Molybdenum helps the body use its stores of iron and assists in the burning of fat for energy. And vanadium may be beneficial for people with diabetes because of its ability to enhance or mimic the effects of the hormone insulin, which regulates blood sugar (glucose) levels.

▼ HOW MUCH YOU NEED

There is no RDA for many trace minerals, because scientific evidence is too scanty to provide a firm requirement. Instead, an Adequate Intake (AI) has been established for some: For manganese, it's 2.3 mg for men and 1.8 mg for women; for fluoride, 4.0 mg for men and 3.0 mg for women; for molybdenum, 45 mcg for both men and women. For boron and vanadium there is no AI; however, a safe upper limit has been set at 20 mg for boron and 1.8 mg for vanadium for both men and women. No RDA or AI has been set for silicon.

IF YOU GET TOO LITTLE
A fluoride deficiency makes people more prone to cavities, and a low boron intake may weaken bones. Deficiencies of manganese, vanadium, and silicon (determined mostly from animal studies) can result in poor growth and development, imbalances in cholesterol levels, and problems making insulin.

IF YOU GET TOO MUCH
In most cases, there is no reason to take high doses of these trace minerals. However, the majority do not cause serious adverse reactions when ingested in large

amounts. Manganese toxicity, which has been noted in people inhaling the metal in mines, can cause severe psychiatric disorders, violent rages, poor coordination, and stiff muscles. Very high doses of boron may produce diarrhea, vomiting, nausea, and fatigue. Too much vanadium can cause cramping, diarrhea, and a green tongue.

▼ HOW TO TAKE IT

DOSAGE
Many bone-building formulas and multivitamin and mineral supplements contain varying doses of trace minerals, including up to 3 mg of boron, 10 mg of manganese, 25 mg of silicon, and 10 mcg of vanadium.

You probably don't need to take individual trace minerals, though single supplements such as manganese (up to 100 mg a day) are available. For most people, a balanced diet plus a high-quality multivitamin/mineral will supply all the needed trace minerals.

GUIDELINES FOR USE
• Boron is probably best taken as part of a bone-building supplement that also contains calcium, manganese, magnesium, and other minerals. Manganese absorption may be impaired by a high iron intake.

▼ OTHER SOURCES

Manganese is present in whole grains, pineapple, nuts, and leafy greens. Nuts and leafy greens also supply boron, as do broccoli, apples, and raisins. Vanadium is found in whole grains, shellfish, mushrooms, soy products, and oats. Silicon is available in whole grains, turnips, beets, and soy products.

SHOPPING HINTS

■ A popular form of vanadium is vanadyl sulfate, which appears to be easy on the stomach and also efficiently absorbed.

■ Some manufacturers claim that manganese picolinate and manganese gluconate are better absorbed than other forms of the mineral, but there's no real evidence to recommend one specific form over another.

■ A substantial and safe natural source of silicon is vegetal silica, an extract of the herb horsetail.

LATEST FINDINGS

■ A manganese-poor diet may raise the risk of heart disease, according to preliminary results of a recent animal study from the University of Maine. Animals lacking this mineral produced less of a substance called glycosaminoglycan, an important component of connective tissue found in arteries. The researchers hypothesize this scenario makes LDL ("bad") cholesterol more likely to accumulate in artery walls.

DID YOU KNOW?

Processed foods, such as white bread, contain less silicon than their whole grain counterparts.

VALERIAN *(Valeriana officinalis)*

It's three o'clock in the morning, and you're wide awake—again. You wish there was something that you could safely take to help you fall asleep. Valerian may be just the natural remedy that you're looking for, because this herb gently induces slumber, without the unpleasant side effects of conventional drugs.

COMMON USES
■ Promotes restful sleep.
■ Soothes stress and anxiety.
■ Improves the symptoms of some digestive disorders.

FORMS
■ Capsule
■ Tablet
■ Softgel
■ Liquid
■ Dried herb/Tea

▼ WHAT IT IS

In Germany, Great Britain, and other European countries, valerian is officially approved as a sleep aid by medical authorities. A perennial plant native to North America and Europe, valerian has pinkish-colored flowers that grow from a tuberous rootstock, or rhizome.

Harvested when the plant is two years old, the rootstock contains a number of important compounds—valepotriates, valeric acid, and volatile oils among them—that at one time or another were each thought to be responsible for the herb's sedative powers. Many experts believe that valerian's effectiveness may be the result of synergy among the various compounds.

▼ WHAT IT DOES

Taken for centuries as an aid to sleep, valerian can also act as a calming agent in stressful daytime situations. It is used in treating anxiety disorders and conditions worsened by stress, such as diverticulosis and irritable bowel syndrome.

MAJOR BENEFITS
Compounds in valerian seem to affect brain receptors for a nerve chemical (neurotransmitter) called gamma-aminobutyric acid, or GABA. It's through this interaction that valerian promotes sleep and eases anxiety.

Unlike benzodiazepines—drugs such as diazepam (Valium) or alprazolam (Xanax) commonly prescribed for these disorders—valerian is not addictive and does not make you feel drugged. Rather than inducing sleep directly, valerian calms the brain and body so sleep can occur naturally. One of the benefits of valerian for insomniacs is that when taken at recommended doses, it doesn't make you feel groggy in the morning as some prescription drugs do.

According to various studies, valerian works as well as prescription drugs for many individuals, and when compared

 ALERT

SIDE EFFECTS
• Studies have shown that even in amounts 20 times higher than recommended, valerian has no dangerous side effects.

• Extremely large doses or long-term use can cause dizziness, restlessness, blurred vision, nausea, headache, giddiness, liver toxicity, and heart problems

CAUTION
• For a time after you take valerian, avoid driving or performing hazardous tasks that require you to be alert and focused.

• Avoid alcohol while taking valerian.

• Because of the risk of excessive drowsiness or disorientation, don't take valerian with prescription tranquilizers or sleeping pills.

• If you are pregnant or breast-feeding, do not use valerian.

• **Reminder:** If you have a medical or psychiatric condition, talk to your doctor before taking supplements.

with a placebo, appears to lull a person to sleep. In one study, 128 people were given one of two valerian preparations or a placebo. It was found that the herb improved sleep quality: Those taking valerian fell asleep more quickly and woke up less often than those receiving a placebo. In another study involving insomniacs, nearly all participants reported improved sleep when taking valerian, and 44% classified their sleep quality as perfect.

Although modern interest in valerian as an anti-anxiety aid is relatively recent, the herb is increasingly recommended by herbalists and nutritionally oriented physicians for this purpose.

ADDITIONAL BENEFITS
Valerian helps relax the smooth muscle of the gastrointestinal tract, making it valuable for the treatment of irritable bowel syndrome and diverticulosis, both of which often involve painful spasms of the intestine. In addition, because flare-ups of these disorders are sometimes triggered by stress, valerian's calming action may also account for its effectiveness.

▼ HOW TO TAKE IT

DOSAGE
For insomnia: Take 250 to 500 mg of the powdered standardized extract in pill form or 1 teaspoon of the liquid extract 30 to 45 minutes before bedtime. Studies show that for most people, higher doses produce no additional benefit. However, if the low dose does not work for you, you can safely use as much as 900 mg (or 2 teaspoons of the liquid extract).
For anxiety: Consume 250 mg twice a day, along with 250 to 500 mg prior to bedtime.

GUIDELINES FOR USE
• If you opt for the liquid extract, try blending it with a little honey or sugar to make this herb, which is a bit unpleasant tasting, more palatable.

• Although valerian is not addictive, it is not a good idea to rely on any substance, herbal or not, to fall asleep every night. Therefore, don't take valerian nightly for more than two weeks in a row.

• Taking valerian with other herbs, such as chamomile, hops, melissa (also known as lemon balm), or passionflower, may increase its effectiveness as a sleep aid. Valerian can also be used with other herbs: with St. John's wort if you're depressed and with kava if you're anxious.

SHOPPING HINTS
■ When buying valerian, look for a product made from a standardized extract that contains 0.8% valeric (or valerenic) acid.

LATEST FINDINGS
■ Prescription sleep aids often cause grogginess the morning after they are taken and can impair a person's ability to drive or perform other tasks requiring concentration. Valerian does not, according to a German study. Researchers compared the effects of valerian; valerian and hops; a benzodiazepine drug; and a placebo. The herbal preparations and the drug all improved sleep quality. The benzodiazepine drug reduced performance the next morning, but the herbs did not. However, performance was slightly impaired for two or three hours after taking the herbs.

DID YOU KNOW?
Valerian preparations have a very disagreeable odor—so much so that inexperienced users may think they have a bad batch. Don't be put off by the smell; it's completely normal.

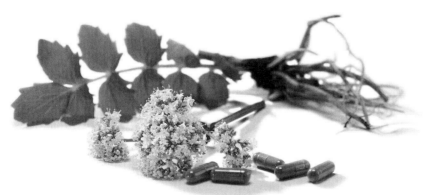

The root of the valerian plant contains compounds that relax the mind and promote sleep.

VITAMIN A

One of the first vitamins to be discovered, this essential nutrient keeps your eyesight keen, your skin healthy, and your immune system strong. And so it follows that an extra dose of vitamin A may help treat various eye problems, a number of skin disorders, and a wide range of infections.

COMMON USES

■ Fights colds, flu, and other types of infections.

■ Treats skin disorders.

■ Heals wounds, burns, and ulcers.

■ Maintains eye health.

■ Enhances chemotherapy.

■ Eases inflammatory bowel disease.

FORMS

■ Tablet

■ Capsule

■ Softgel

■ Liquid

▼ WHAT IT IS

Vitamin A, a fat-soluble nutrient, is stored in the liver. The body gets part of its vitamin A from animal fats and makes part in the intestine from beta-carotene and other carotenoids in fruits and vegetables. Vitamin A is present in the body in various chemical forms called retinoids—so named because the vitamin is essential to the health of the retina of the eye.

▼ WHAT IT DOES

This vitamin prevents night blindness; maintains the skin and cells that line the respiratory and gastrointestinal tracts; and helps build healthy teeth and bones. It is vital for normal reproduction, growth, and development too. In addition, vitamin A is crucial to the immune system, including the plentiful supply of immune cells that line the airways and digestive tract and form an important line of defense against infectious disease.

MAJOR BENEFITS

Vitamin A is perhaps best known for its ability to maintain vision, especially night vision, assisting the eye in adjusting from bright light to darkness. It can also alleviate such specific eye complaints as "dry eye," in addition to its many other benefits.

By boosting immunity, vitamin A greatly strengthens resistance to infections, including sore throat, colds, flu, and bronchitis. It may also combat cold sores and shingles (caused by a herpes virus), warts (a viral skin infection), eye infections, and vaginal yeast infections—and perhaps even control bothersome allergies.

The vitamin may help the immune system battle against breast and lung cancers and improve survival rates in those with leukemia; in addition, animal studies suggest it inhibits melanoma, an often deadly form of skin cancer. Another benefit for cancer patients is that vitamin A may possibly enhance the effectiveness of chemotherapy.

ADDITIONAL BENEFITS

Vitamin A was first used in the 1940s to treat skin disorders, including acne and psoriasis, but the doses were high and toxic. Scientists later developed

ALERT

CAUTION

• Like vitamin D (another fat-soluble vitamin), vitamin A can build up to toxic levels, so be careful not to get too much.

• If you're pregnant or considering pregnancy, don't take more than 5,000 IU of vitamin A daily; higher doses may cause birth defects. Practice effective birth control when taking doses higher than 5,000 IU and for at least a month afterward.

• **Reminder:** If you have a medical condition, talk to your doctor before taking supplements.

safer vitamin A derivatives (notably retinoic acid); now sold as prescription drugs, these include the acne and anti-wrinkle cream Retin-A. Lower doses of vitamin A (25,000 IU a day) can be used to treat a range of skin conditions, including acne, dry skin, eczema, rosacea, and psoriasis. Vitamin A also promotes healing of skin wounds and can be applied to cuts, scrapes, and burns; it may hasten recovery from sprains and strains.

The therapeutic effects of vitamin A extend to the lining of the digestive tract, where it helps treat inflammatory bowel disease and ulcers. In addition, getting enough of this vitamin will speed recovery in people who have had a stroke. Women with heavy or prolonged menstrual periods are sometimes deficient in this vitamin, so supplements may be of value in treating this condition as well.

▼ HOW MUCH YOU NEED

The RDA for vitamin A is 2,300 IU a day for adult women (over age 19), and 3,000 IU a day for adult men (over age 19).

IF YOU GET TOO LITTLE
Although quite rare in the United States, a vitamin A deficiency can cause night blindness (even total blindness) and a greatly lowered resistance to infection. Milder cases of deficiency do occur, especially in the elderly, who often have vitamin-poor diets. Infections such as pneumonia can deplete vitamin A stores.

IF YOU GET TOO MUCH
An overabundance of vitamin A can be a real problem. A single dose of 500,000 IU may induce weakness and

vomiting. And 25,000 IU a day for six years has been reported to cause serious liver disease (cirrhosis). Signs of toxicity include dry, cracking skin and brittle nails, hair that falls out easily, bleeding gums, weight loss, irritability, fatigue, and nausea.

▼ HOW TO TAKE IT

DOSAGE
Multivitamins supply vitamin A, often in the form of beta-carotene. For specific complaints in adults, up to 10,000 IU a day is generally safe for long-term use (except for pregnant women and those considering pregnancy, who should not exceed 5,000 IU a day).

As a broad guideline, it's safe to take 25,000 IU a day for up to a month or 100,000 IU for up to a week, though in some cases higher doses may be needed for specific conditions.

GUIDELINES FOR USE
• Take supplements with food; a little fat in the diet aids absorption.

• Vitamin E and zinc help the body use vitamin A, which in turn boosts absorption of iron from foods.

▼ OTHER SOURCES

Vitamin A is richly represented in fish, egg yolks, butter, organ meats such as liver (3 ounces provide more than 9,000 IU), and fortified milk (check the label to be sure). Dark green, yellow, orange, and red fruits and vegetables have large amounts of beta-carotene and many other carotenoids, which the body makes into vitamin A on an as-needed basis.

FACTS & TIPS
■ You can't overdose on vitamin A by eating carotenoid-rich fruits and vegetables, such as apricots, leafy greens, or cantaloupe. Although your body converts some carotenoids to vitamin A, it makes only as much as it needs. Unless you eat a lot of liver or oily fish, it's almost impossible to get too much vitamin A from your diet.

■ Vitamin A doses can be given as retinol equivalents (RE) rather than international units (IU). One RE is equivalent to 3.3 IU.

LATEST FINDINGS
■ Vitamin A shows promise in the treatment of diabetes. In two recent studies, up to 25,000 IU of vitamin A daily improved insulin's ability to control blood sugar. (Poor blood sugar control is a prime problem in people with diabetes.)

■ A Brazilian study found vitamin A may combat chronic lung diseases. After 30 days of taking supplements, men who received 5,000 IU a day could breathe better than those given a placebo.

DID YOU KNOW?
You'd have to eat more than 10 large eggs to meet the daily RDA for vitamin A. Most people get enough from other animal sources and from carotenoid-rich fruits and vegetables.

VITAMIN B$_6$

This remarkable nutrient is probably involved in more bodily processes than any other vitamin or mineral. Government surveys indicate, however, that one-third of all adults—and half of all women—are not getting enough B$_6$ in their diets. In addition, this vitamin seems to play a role in treating PMS, asthma, and carpal tunnel syndrome.

COMMON USES

- Helps prevent cardiovascular disease and strokes.
- Helps to lift depression.
- Eases insomnia.
- Treats carpal tunnel syndrome.
- May lessen PMS symptoms.
- Helps relieve asthma attacks.

FORMS

- Tablet
- Capsule
- Liquid
- Powder

▼ WHAT IT IS

Vitamin B$_6$, unequivocally the "workhorse" of nutrients, performs more than 100 jobs innumerable times a day. It functions primarily as a coenzyme, a substance that acts in concert with enzymes to speed up chemical reactions in the cells.

Another name for vitamin B$_6$ is pyridoxine. In supplement form, it is available as pyridoxine hydrochloride or pyridoxal-5-phosphate (P-5-P). Either form satisfies most needs, but some nutritionally oriented physicians prefer P-5-P because it may be better absorbed.

▼ WHAT IT DOES

Forming red blood cells, helping cells make proteins, manufacturing brain chemicals (neurotransmitters) such as serotonin, and releasing stored forms of energy are just a few of the functions of vitamin B$_6$. There is also evidence that vitamin B$_6$ plays a role in preventing and treating many diseases.

PREVENTION

Getting enough B$_6$ through the diet or supplements may help prevent heart disease. Working with folic acid and vitamin B$_{12}$, this vitamin assists the body in processing homocysteine, an amino acid-like compound that has been linked to an increased risk of heart disease and other vascular disorders when large amounts are present in the blood.

ADDITIONAL BENEFITS

Some women suffering from premenstrual syndrome (PMS) report that vitamin B$_6$ provides relief from many of the symptoms. This beneficial effect probably occurs because of the vitamin's involvement in clearing excess estrogen from the body.

And in its role as a building block for neurotransmitters, vitamin B$_6$ may be useful in reducing the likelihood of having epileptic seizures, as well as lifting depression. In fact, up to 25% of people with depression may be deficient in vitamin B$_6$.

In addition, the vitamin maintains nerve health. People with diabetes, who are at risk for nerve damage, can also benefit from B$_6$. Furthermore, it is effective in easing the symptoms of

---

 ALERT

CAUTION

- Long-term use of high doses of B$_6$ may cause nerve damage. Stop taking the supplement and call your doctor if you develop any new numbness or tingling.

- Because of the risk of unwanted reactions, consult your doctor before taking a vitamin B$_6$ supplement if you also take an anticonvulsant medication or the prescription drug levodopa for Parkinson's disease.

- **Reminder:** If you have a medical or psychiatric condition, talk to your doctor before taking supplements.

carpal tunnel syndrome, which involves nerve inflammation in the wrist. And for people with asthma, vitamin B_6 may reduce the intensity and frequency of attacks; it is especially important for those people who are taking the asthma drug theophylline.

▼ HOW MUCH YOU NEED

The RDA for vitamin B_6 is 1.3 mg a day for women and men younger than age 50; it's 1.5 mg a day for women older than age 50, and 1.7 mg a day for men older than age 50. Therapeutic doses are usually higher.

IF YOU GET TOO LITTLE
A recent survey found that half of all American women fail to meet the RDA for vitamin B_6. Women taking oral contraceptives may have especially low levels of this vitamin. Mild deficiencies of vitamin B_6 can raise homocysteine levels, increasing the risk of heart and vascular diseases.

Symptoms of severe deficiency, which is rare, are skin disorders such as dermatitis, sores around the mouth, and acne. Neurological signs include insomnia, depression, and in really extreme cases, seizures and brain wave abnormalities.

IF YOU GET TOO MUCH
High doses of vitamin B_6 (more than 2,000 mg a day) can cause nerve damage when taken for long periods. In rare cases, prolonged use at lower doses (200 to 300 mg a day) can have the same consequence. Fortunately, nerve damage is completely reversible once you discontinue the vitamin. If you're using B_6 for nerve pain, and if you experience any new numbness or tingling, stop taking the vitamin and call your doctor. Doses up to 100 mg a day are safe, even for long-term use.

▼ HOW TO TAKE IT

DOSAGE
You can keep homocysteine levels in check with just 3 mg of B_6 a day, but a daily dose of 50 mg is often recommended. Higher doses are needed for therapeutic uses.

For PMS: Take 100 mg of B_6 a day.
For acute carpal tunnel syndrome: Take 50 mg of B_6 or P-5-P three times a day.
For asthma: Take 50 mg of B_6 twice a day.

GUIDELINES FOR USE
• Vitamin B_6 is best absorbed in doses of no more than 100 mg at one time. When taking higher doses, this more gradual intake will also decrease your chances of nerve damage.

▼ OTHER SOURCES

Fish, poultry, meats, chickpeas, potatoes, avocados, and bananas are all good sources of vitamin B_6.

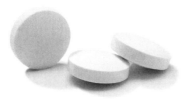

FACTS & TIPS
■ Vitamin B_6 supplements can relieve morning sickness in pregnant women. Though the vitamin appears to be safe in the dosages typically recommended (25 mg a day), there have been no studies showing how extra vitamin B_6 may affect the developing baby. Women who are troubled by morning sickness should check with their doctor before taking B_6.

LATEST FINDINGS
■ A lack of vitamin B_6 may cause stress, anxiety, and depression, according to a study of men participating in a bereavement group. Men with low levels of B_6 were more distressed and anxious than those with adequate levels. Researchers said that an effective depression treatment may begin with vitamin B_6 supplements rather than antidepressant drugs, which can have side effects.

■ Vitamin B_6 may protect against heart disease—and not just because it lowers levels of the risk-increasing amino acid-like substance homocysteine. One study of 1,550 people from 19 European clinics found that those who placed in the bottom fifth of the group in terms of vitamin B_6 levels had twice the risk of heart disease, regardless of their homocysteine levels.

DID YOU KNOW?
You'd have to eat 74 bananas to get the amount of vitamin B_6 in a single 50 mg supplement pill.

VITAMIN B$_{12}$

Although this vitamin is plentiful in most people's diets, after the age of 50 some individuals have only a limited ability to absorb B$_{12}$ from food. Supplements are usually recommended, because mild deficiencies may increase the risk of heart disease, depression, and possibly even Alzheimer's disease.

COMMON USES

- Prevents a form of anemia.
- Helps reduce depression.
- Thwarts nerve pain, numbness, and tingling.
- Lowers the risk of heart disease.
- May improve multiple sclerosis and tinnitus (ringing in the ears).

FORMS

- Tablet
- Capsule
- Lozenge

▼ WHAT IT IS

Also known as cobalamin, vitamin B$_{12}$ was the last vitamin to be discovered. In the late 1940s it was identified as the substance in calf's liver that cured pernicious anemia, a potentially fatal disease primarily affecting older adults.

Vitamin B$_{12}$ is the only B vitamin the body stores in large amounts, mostly in the liver. The body absorbs B$_{12}$ through a very complicated process: Digestive enzymes in the presence of enough stomach acid separate B$_{12}$ from the protein in foods. The vitamin then binds with a substance called intrinsic factor (a protein produced by cells in the stomach lining) before being carried to the small intestine, where it is absorbed.

Low levels of stomach acid or an inadequate amount of intrinsic factor—both of which occur with age—can lead to deficiencies. However, because the body has good reserves of B$_{12}$, it can take several years for a shortfall to develop.

▼ WHAT IT DOES

Vitamin B$_{12}$ is essential for cell replication and is particularly important for red blood cell production. It maintains the protective sheath around nerves (myelin), assists in converting food to energy, and plays a critical role in the production of DNA and RNA, the genetic material in cells.

PREVENTION

Moderately high blood levels of homocysteine, an amino acid-like substance, have been linked to an increased risk of heart disease. Working with folic acid, vitamin B$_{12}$ helps the body process homocysteine and so may lower that risk.

Because of its beneficial effects on the nerves, vitamin B$_{12}$ may help prevent a number of neurological disorders, as well as the numbness and tingling often associated with diabetes. It may also play a part in treating depression.

ADDITIONAL BENEFITS

Research shows that low levels of B$_{12}$ are common in people with Alzheimer's disease. Whether this deficiency is a contributing factor to the disease or simply a result of it is unknown.

The nutrient does, however, keep the immune system healthy. Some studies suggest that it lengthens the amount of time between infection with the HIV virus and the development of AIDS.

 ALERT

CAUTION

- If you take a vitamin B$_{12}$ supplement, you must also have a folic acid supplement: A high intake of one can mask a deficiency of the other.

- Excessive alcohol hinders absorption of vitamin B$_{12}$.

- **Reminder:** If you have a medical or psychiatric condition, talk to your doctor before taking supplements.

Other research indicates adequate B_{12} intake improves immune responses in older people.

With its beneficial effect on nerves, vitamin B_{12} may lessen ringing in the ears (tinnitus). As a component of myelin, it is valuable in treating multiple sclerosis, a disease that involves the destruction of this nerve covering. And through its role in cell replication, B_{12} may improve symptoms of rosacea.

▼ HOW MUCH YOU NEED

The RDA for vitamin B_{12} is 2.4 mcg a day for adults. But, many experts recommend that you get 100 to 400 mcg. Supplements of vitamin B_{12} are very important for older people and vegans (who eat no meat products).

IF YOU GET TOO LITTLE

Symptoms of a vitamin B_{12} deficiency include fatigue, depression, numbness and tingling in the extremities caused by nerve damage, muscle weakness, confusion, and memory loss. Dementia and pernicious anemia can develop; both are reversible if caught early.

The level of vitamin B_{12} in the blood decreases with age. Individuals with ulcers, Crohn's disease, or other gastrointestinal disorders are at risk for B_{12} deficiencies, as are those taking prescription medication for epilepsy (seizures), chronic heartburn, or gout.

IF YOU GET TOO MUCH

Excess vitamin B_{12} is readily excreted in urine; there are no known adverse effects from a high intake of B_{12}.

▼ HOW TO TAKE IT

DOSAGE

A typical multiple vitamin usually contains between 50 and 100 mcg of vitamin B_{12}, which is sufficient to prevent a B_{12} deficiency. However, a general dose of 1,000 mcg of vitamin B_{12} a day is useful for heart disease prevention, pernicious anemia, numbness and tingling, tinnitus, multiple sclerosis, and rosacea.

If blood tests show you're deficient in B_{12}, it may be that you are not producing enough intrinsic factor and B_{12} shots or a prescription nasal spray may be necessary; ask your doctor.

GUIDELINES FOR USE

• Take vitamin B_{12} once a day, preferably in the morning, along with at least 400 mcg of folic acid.

• Most multivitamins contain at least the RDA of vitamin B_{12} and folic acid; B-complex supplements have higher amounts. For larger, therapeutic amounts, look for a supplement with just vitamin B_{12} or B_{12} with folic acid.

• Using a sublingual (under-the-tongue) form enhances absorption.

▼ OTHER SOURCES

Animal foods are the primary source of B_{12}. These include organ meats, oysters, sardines and other fish, eggs, meat, and cheese. Brewer's yeast is another source. Some breakfast cereals are fortified with this vitamin as well.

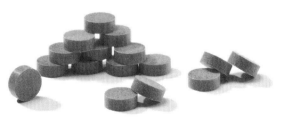

FACTS & TIPS

■ As many as 20% of older people may be deficient in vitamin B_{12}, and most have no symptoms. As people age, they can develop atrophic gastritis, which reduces stomach acid production. Without enough acid, the body cannot separate vitamin B_{12} from the protein in foods. However, the body can absorb enough B_{12} from supplements or fortified breakfast cereal, forms in which the vitamin doesn't have to be separated from protein.

LATEST FINDINGS

■ Having a sufficient amount of vitamin B_{12} in the body may slow the progression of HIV infection to AIDS, according to a study of 310 HIV-positive men. On average, those with low B_{12} levels developed AIDS within four years of the start of the study, versus eight years in men who had higher B_{12} levels.

■ Older people with mildly low vitamin B_{12} levels may not get the full protection of a pneumonia vaccine. In a study of 30 elderly people, those with inadequate B_{12} stores produced fewer antibodies to the pneumonia virus after vaccination than those with sufficient levels of B_{12}. This would reduce their ability to fight off the disease.

DID YOU KNOW?

You would have to eat 5 ounces of Swiss cheese to meet the RDA for B_{12}—and 125 pounds to get a therapeutic dose of this vitamin.

VITAMIN C

This vitamin is probably better known and more widely used than any other nutritional supplement sold in the United States today. But even if you think you're familiar with vitamin C, read on. You may be quite surprised to discover exactly how versatile and health-enhancing this popular nutrient truly is.

COMMON USES

- Enhances immunity.
- Minimizes cold symptoms; shortens duration of illness.
- Speeds wound healing.
- Promotes healthy gums.
- Treats asthma.
- Helps prevent cataracts.
- Protects against some forms of cancer and heart disease.

FORMS

- Tablet
- Capsule
- Liquid
- Powder

▼ WHAT IT IS

As early as 1742 lemon juice was known to prevent scurvy, a disease that plagued long-distance sailors. But not until 1928 was the healthful component in lemon juice identified as vitamin C. And its anti-scurvy, or anti-scorbutic, effect is the root of vitamin C's scientific name: ascorbic acid.

Today, interest in vitamin C is based less on its ability to cure scurvy than on its potential to protect cells. As the body's primary water-soluble antioxidant, vitamin C helps fight damage caused by unstable oxygen molecules called free radicals–especially in those areas that are mostly water, such as the interior of cells.

▼ WHAT IT DOES

Vitamin C is active throughout the body. It helps strengthen the capillaries (the tiniest blood vessels) and cell walls and is crucial for the formation of collagen (a protein found in connective tissue). In these ways, vitamin C prevents bruising, promotes healing, and keeps ligaments (which connect muscle to bone), tendons (which connect bone to bone), and gums strong and healthy. It also aids in producing hemoglobin in red blood cells and assists the body in absorbing iron from foods.

PREVENTION

As an antioxidant, vitamin C offers protection against cancer and heart disease; several studies have shown that low levels of this vitamin are linked to heart attacks.

In addition, vitamin C may actually lengthen life. In one study, men who consumed more than 300 mg of vitamin C a day (from food and supplements) lived longer than men who consumed less than 50 mg a day.

Another study found that over the long term, vitamin C supplements protect against cataracts, a clouding of the eye's lens that interferes with vision. Women who took vitamin C for 10 years or more had a 77% lower rate of early "lens opacities," the beginning stage of cataracts, than women who didn't take vitamin C.

ALERT

SIDE EFFECTS
- Large amounts of vitamin C (more than 2,000 mg a day) can cause loose stools, diarrhea, and gas; if such reactions occur, lower your dose.

CAUTION
- There is some evidence that megadoses of vitamin C can actually increase cell damage rather than help to prevent it. Lower your dose to recommended levels and consult your doctor if you have any concerns.

- Don't take more than 500 mg a day if you have kidney disease or hemochromatosis, a genetic tendency to store excess iron (vitamin C enhances iron absorption).

- Vitamin C can distort the accuracy of medical tests for diabetes, colon cancer, and hemoglobin levels. Let your doctor know if you're taking it.

- **Reminder:** If you have a medical condition, talk to your doctor before taking supplements.

ADDITIONAL BENEFITS

Does vitamin C prevent colds? Probably not, but it can help lessen symptoms and may shorten the duration of this illness. In a 1995 analysis of studies that explored the connection between vitamin C and colds, the researchers concluded that taking 1,000 to 6,000 mg a day at the onset of cold symptoms reduced its duration by 21%, about one day. Other studies have shown that vitamin C helps elderly patients fight severe respiratory infections.

Vitamin C also appears to be a natural antihistamine. High doses of the vitamin can block the effect of inflammatory substances produced by the body in response to pollen, pet dander, or other allergens.

This nutrient is an effective asthma remedy as well. Numerous studies have found that vitamin C in supplement form helped prevent or improve asthmatic symptoms.

For people with type 1 diabetes, which interferes with the transport of vitamin C into cells, supplementing with 1,000 to 3,000 mg a day may prevent complications of the disease, such as eye problems and high cholesterol levels.

▼ HOW MUCH YOU NEED

The RDA for vitamin C for men is 90 mg a day and for women, 75 mg (smokers need an additional 35 mg). But even conservative experts think an optimal intake is at least 200 mg a day, and they recommend higher doses for the treatment of specific diseases.

IF YOU GET TOO LITTLE

You'd have to consume less than 10 mg a day to get scurvy, but receiving less than 50 mg of vitamin C a day has been linked with an increased risk of heart attack, cataracts, and a shorter life.

IF YOU GET TOO MUCH

Large doses of vitamin C—more than 2,000 mg a day—can cause loose stools, diarrhea, gas, and bloating; all can be corrected by reducing your daily dose. At this level, the vitamin may interfere with the absorption of copper and selenium, so be sure you consume enough of these minerals in foods or supplements.

▼ HOW TO TAKE IT

DOSAGE

For general health: Get 500 mg of vitamin C a day through foods and supplements.
For the treatment of various diseases: Depending on the condition, about 1,000 mg a day may be appropriate for lessening symptoms.

GUIDELINES FOR USE

• Vitamin C is best taken with meals.

• Experts recommend taking the vitamin in combination with other antioxidants, such as vitamin E and flavonoids. This helps with absorption and enables the body to recycle its antioxidants, minimizing risks associated with taking high doses of a single antioxidant.

▼ OTHER SOURCES

Citrus fruits and juices, broccoli, red peppers, dark greens, strawberries, and kiwifruits are all good sources of vitamin C.

SHOPPING HINTS

■ Don't spend extra money on specialized vitamin C products (such as esterified C). There's no evidence that they are more efficiently absorbed than plain old ascorbic acid.

LATEST FINDINGS

■ Vitamin C may help prevent reblockage (restenosis) of arteries after angioplasty (an alternative to bypass surgery). A study of 119 angioplasty patients found that restenosis occurred in just 24% of those who took 500 mg of vitamin C a day for four months, compared with 43% of those who did not take the vitamin.

■ In addition to being an antioxidant, vitamin C helps the body recycle other antioxidants. In one study, vitamin E concentrations were 18% higher in those who got more than 220 mg of vitamin C a day, compared with people who got 120 mg or less.

DID YOU KNOW?

An 8-ounce glass of fresh-squeezed orange juice supplies 124 mg of vitamin C—more than twice the RDA for this vitamin.

VITAMIN D

Commonly called the sunshine vitamin (because your body makes all it needs when you're exposed to enough sunlight), vitamin D is essential for bone health and may slow the progression of arthritis. It is also believed to strengthen the immune system and possibly prevent some cancers.

COMMON USES

- Aids in the body's absorption of calcium.
- Promotes healthy bones.
- Strengthens teeth.
- May protect against some types of cancer.

FORMS

- Tablet
- Capsule
- Softgel
- Liquid

▼ WHAT IT IS

Technically a hormone, vitamin D is produced within the body when the skin is exposed to the ultraviolet B (UVB) rays in sunlight. Theoretically, spending a few minutes in the sun each day supplies all the vitamin D your body needs, but many people don't get enough sun to generate adequate vitamin D, especially in the winter.

What's more, the body's ability to manufacture vitamin D declines with age, so vitamin D deficiencies are common in older people. But even young adults may not have sufficient vitamin D stores.

One study of nearly 300 patients (of all ages) hospitalized for a variety of causes found that 57% of them did not have high enough levels of vitamin D. Of particular concern was the observation that a vitamin D deficiency was present in a third of the people who obtained the recommended amount of vitamin D through diet or supplements.

This finding suggests that current recommendations for vitamin D may not be high enough.

▼ WHAT IT DOES

The basic function of vitamin D is to regulate blood levels of calcium and phosphorus, helping to build strong bones and healthy teeth.

PREVENTION

Studies have shown that vitamin D is important in the prevention of osteoporosis, a disease that causes porous bones and thus an increased risk of fractures. Without sufficient vitamin D, the body cannot absorb calcium from food or supplements—no matter how much calcium you consume. When blood calcium levels are low, the body will move calcium from the bones to the blood to supply the muscles—especially the heart—and the nerves with the amount they need. Over time, this reallocation of calcium leads to a loss of bone mass.

ADDITIONAL BENEFITS

Scientists are continuing to discover more about the functions of vitamin D in the body. Some studies suggest that it is important for a healthy immune system. Others indicate that it may help prevent prostate, colon, or breast cancer.

The results of one study showed that adequate vitamin D slowed the

 ALERT

CAUTION

- Overuse of vitamin D supplements can result in elevated blood levels of calcium, leading to weight loss, nausea, and heart and kidney damage.

- Avoid taking vitamin D supplements with magnesium-containing antacids or with thiazide diuretics (Indapamide, Hydrochlorothiazide, and others).

- **Reminder:** If you have a medical condition, talk to your doctor before taking supplements.

progression of osteoarthritis in the knees, although it did not prevent the disease from developing initially.

▼ HOW MUCH YOU NEED

The government-established level of intake (called AI, or Adequate Intake) sufficient to maintain healthy blood levels of vitamin D is 200 IU a day for people 50 or under; 400 IU for those ages 51 to 70; and 600 IU for those over age 70. Many experts, however, think the recommendations for people over age 50 are too low.

IF YOU GET TOO LITTLE

A vitamin D deficiency can harm the bones, causing a bone-weakening disease in children (rickets) and increasing the risk of osteoporosis in adults. A deficiency can also cause diarrhea, insomnia, nervousness, and muscle twitches. The likelihood of a child developing rickets today is remote, however, because vitamin D is added to milk. In addition, children typically spend enough time in the sunshine to generate ample vitamin D.

IF YOU GET TOO MUCH

Although your body effectively rids itself of any extra vitamin D it makes from sunlight, overloading on supplements may create problems. Daily doses of 1,000 to 2,000 IU over six months can cause constipation or diarrhea, headache, loss of appetite, nausea and vomiting, heartbeat irregularities, and extreme fatigue. Continued high doses weaken the bones and allow calcium to accumulate in soft tissues, such as the muscles.

▼ HOW TO TAKE IT

DOSAGE

As little as 10 to 15 minutes of midday sunlight on your face, hands, and arms two or three times a week can supply all the vitamin D you need.

But if you are over age 50; if you don't drink milk (which is fortified with vitamin D); if you don't get outdoors much between the hours of 8 A.M. and 3 P.M.; or if you always wear sunscreen, you might want to consider taking vitamin D supplements.

Many experts recommend 400 to 600 IU a day for people over age 50 and 800 IU for those over age 70; 200 to 400 IU a day is probably sufficient for younger adults.

GUIDELINES FOR USE

• Supplements can be taken at any time of day, with or without food.

• Most daily multivitamins contain up to 400 IU of vitamin D. It is also often found in calcium supplements.

▼ OTHER SOURCES

Vitamin D is added to milk; one cup contains 100 IU. Some breakfast cereals are fortified with 40 to 100 IU of vitamin D in each serving. Fatty fish, such as herring, salmon, and tuna, are naturally rich in the vitamin.

FACTS & TIPS

■ In northern latitudes, the sun's rays aren't strong enough to stimulate vitamin D production in the winter. People affected are those above the 42°N latitude (in Boston or Chicago) from November to February and those above the 40°N latitude (Philadelphia, Denver) in January and February. If you get sufficient sun the rest of the year, your body can store enough vitamin D to carry you to spring. If you don't, consider taking a daily vitamin D supplement in the winter.

■ The milk used to make yogurt, cheese, and other dairy products isn't fortified with vitamin D, so these foods contain only trace amounts of the vitamin.

LATEST FINDINGS

■ Calcium and vitamin D supplements slowed bone loss and reduced the incidence of fractures in 176 men and 213 women over age 65 participating in a recent study. They took 500 mg of calcium and 700 IU of vitamin D a day for three years.

■ Vitamin D may help prevent colon cancer. A study of 438 men found that those with colon cancer had lower blood levels of vitamin D than those who didn't have the disease. Over all, men with the highest vitamin D intake had the best chance of avoiding colon cancer. More study is needed to confirm this finding and to see if the risk is the same for women.

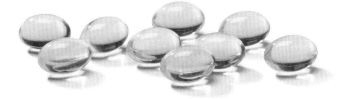

VITAMIN E

A superstar nutrient with much-touted antioxidant capabilities, vitamin E offers a multitude of preventive benefits, including protection against heart disease, cancer, eye problems, and a broad range of other disorders. Working at the body's cellular level, vitamin E may even slow the aging process.

COMMON USES

■ Helps protect against heart disease, certain cancers, and various other chronic ailments.

■ May delay or prevent cataracts.

■ Enhances the immune system.

■ Protects against secondhand smoke and other pollutants.

■ Aids in skin healing.

FORMS

■ Capsule

■ Tablet

■ Softgel

■ Cream

■ Oil

■ Liquid

▼ WHAT IT IS

Vitamin E is a generic term for a group of related compounds called toco-pherols, which occur in four major forms: alpha-, beta-, delta-, and gamma-tocopherols. Alpha-tocopherol is the most common and most potent form of the vitamin. Because it is fat-soluble, vitamin E is stored for relatively long periods in the body, mainly in fat tissue and the liver.

Vitamin E is found in only a few foods, and many of these are high in fat, which makes it difficult to get the amount of vitamin E you require while on a healthy low-fat diet. Therefore, supplements can be very useful in obtaining optimal amounts of this nutrient.

▼ WHAT IT DOES

One of vitamin E's basic functions is to protect cell membranes. It also helps the body use selenium and vitamin K. But vitamin E's current reputation comes from its disease-fighting potential as an antioxidant—meaning it assists in destroying or neutralizing free radicals, the unstable oxygen molecules that cause damage to cells.

PREVENTION

By safeguarding cell membranes and acting as an antioxidant, vitamin E may play a role in preventing cancer. Some of the most compelling research to date suggests that vitamin E can help protect against cardiovascular disease, including heart attack and stroke, by reducing the harmful effects of LDL ("bad") cholesterol and by preventing blood clots.

In addition, vitamin E may offer protection because it works to reduce inflammatory processes that have been linked to heart disease. Findings from two large studies suggest that vitamin E may reduce the risk of heart disease by 25% to 50%—and it may prevent chest pain (angina) as well. And recent findings suggest that taking vitamin E with vitamin C may help block some of the harmful effects of a fatty meal.

ADDITIONAL BENEFITS

Because it protects cells from free-radical damage, some experts think that vitamin E may retard the aging process. There is also evidence to suggest that it improves immune function in the elderly, combats toxins from

ALERT

CAUTION

• Always tell your doctor that you are taking vitamin E supplements.

• People on prescription blood-thinning drugs (anticoagulants) or daily aspirin should consult their doctor before using vitamin E.

• Because of the risk of abnormal bleeding, do not take vitamin E two days before or after elective surgery.

• **Reminder:** If you have a medical condition, talk to your doctor before taking supplements.

cigarette smoke and other pollutants, treats Parkinson's disease, postpones the development of cataracts, and slows the progression of Alzheimer's disease.

Other research found that vitamin E can relieve the severe leg pain caused by a circulatory problem called intermittent claudication. It may alleviate premenstrual breast pain and tenderness as well. In addition, many people report that applying creams or oils containing vitamin E to skin wounds helps promote healing.

▼ HOW MUCH YOU NEED

The RDA for vitamin E is 15 mg (in the form of alpha-tocopherol) for all adults over age 19—which is equal to 22 IU of d-alpha tocopherol (natural E) or 33 IU of dl-alpha tocopherol (the synthetic form found in supplements and some fortified foods). Although this amount may be enough to prevent deficiency, higher doses are needed to provide the full antioxidant effect.

IF YOU GET TOO LITTLE
Intakes of vitamin E below the RDA can lead to neurological damage and shorten the life of red blood cells. If you are eating a balanced diet, however, you are probably not at risk.

IF YOU GET TOO MUCH
No toxic effects from large doses of vitamin E have been discovered, although too much can raise the risk of bleeding. Minor effects, such as headaches and diarrhea, have rarely been reported. Large doses of vitamin E can interfere with the absorption of vitamin A.

The maximum amount considered safe by government standards (the Tolerable Upper Limit) is 1,000 mg (equal to 1,500 IU of natural vitamin E or 1,200 IU of dl-alpha tocopherol, synthetic vitamin E).

▼ HOW TO TAKE IT

DOSAGE
To obtain the disease-fighting potential of vitamin E, many experts recommend 400 to 800 IU daily in capsule or tablet form. (This total includes amounts you get in a multivitamin.) Vitamin E may be particularly effective when taken with vitamin C.

GUIDELINES FOR USE
• Try to take vitamin E supplements at the same time each day. Combining it with a meal decreases stomach irritation and increases the absorption of this fat-soluble vitamin.

• Experts recommend taking the vitamin in combination with other antioxidants, such as vitamin C. This helps with absorption and enables the body to recycle its antioxidants, minimizing risks associated with taking high doses of a single antioxidant.

• For topical use, break open a capsule and apply the oil directly to your skin, or use a commercial cream containing vitamin E as needed.

▼ OTHER SOURCES

Wheat germ is an outstanding dietary source of vitamin E: 1 ounce (about 2 tablespoons) contains the equivalent of 54 IU. Beneficial amounts of vitamin E are also found in vegetable oils, nuts and seeds (hazelnuts, almonds, sunflower seeds), green leafy vegetables, and whole grains.

SHOPPING HINTS
■ Although alpha-tocopherol is the most clinically studied form of vitamin E, there's evidence that the natural form ("d") may be even better. This is because the natural form contains a mixture of tocopherols while the synthetic ("dl") only contains alpha. The only way to get the mixture is to take the natural vitamin E.

LATEST FINDINGS
■ In a recent study of thousands of smokers, vitamin E supplements reduced the risk of prostate cancer by 33% and the death rate from the disease by 41%. The dosage was 50 IU a day, indicating that even low doses of vitamin E may offer protective benefits.

■ Taking vitamin E supplements may strengthen the immune systems of older people. In a study of 88 healthy subjects age 65 and older, those taking 200 IU of vitamin E each day showed the greatest increase in immune-system responses (such as a buildup of antibodies to fight disease).

DID YOU KNOW?
You'd have to eat 4 pounds of hazelnuts or 245 tablespoons of mayonnaise to get the vitamin E supplied by one 400 IU capsule.

VITAMIN K

Doctors have long used vitamin K, which promotes blood clotting, to help heal incisions in surgical patients and to prevent bleeding problems in newborns. This vitamin also aids in building strong bones and may be useful for combating the threat of brittle-bone disease (or osteoporosis) in older women.

COMMON USES

- Reduces the risk of internal hemorrhaging.
- Protects against bleeding problems after surgery.
- Helps build strong bones and ward off or treat osteoporosis.

FORMS

- Tablet
- Liquid

▼ WHAT IT IS

In the 1930s Danish researchers noted that baby chickens fed a fat-free diet developed bleeding problems. They eventually solved the problem with an alfalfa-based compound that they named vitamin K, for Koagulation.

Scientists now know that most of the body's vitamin K needs are met by bacteria in the intestines that produce this vitamin, and only about 20% comes from foods. Deficiencies are rare in healthy people, even though the body doesn't store vitamin K in high amounts.

Natural forms of vitamin K come from chlorophyll—the same substance that gives plants such as alfalfa their green color. Synthetic vitamin K supplements are also available by prescription. Other names for vitamin K are phytonadione and menadiol.

▼ WHAT IT DOES

This single nutrient sets in motion the entire blood-clotting process as soon as a wound occurs. Without it, we might bleed to death. Researchers have discovered vitamin K plays a protective role in bone health as well.

PREVENTION

Doctors often recommend preventive doses of vitamin K if bleeding or hemorrhaging is a concern. Even when no deficiency exists, surgeons frequently order vitamin K before an operation to reduce the risk of postoperative bleeding. Under medical supervision, vitamin K can also be prescribed for excessive menstrual bleeding.

Though not yet a widely accepted treatment, vitamin K may provide great benefits for those suffering from osteoporosis. Some studies show it helps the body make use of calcium and decreases the risk of fractures. Vitamin K may be especially important for bone health in older women. Not surprisingly, it is included among the ingredients in many bone-building formulas.

ADDITIONAL BENEFITS

Vitamin K may play a role in cancer prevention and help those undergoing radiation therapy. Recent findings also put vitamin K in the arsenal of heart-smart nutrients: Some evidence suggests it may halt the buildup of disease-causing plaque in arteries

ALERT

CAUTION

- Supplemental vitamin K (more than is found in a multivitamin) should be taken only with your doctor's consent.

- High doses of vitamin E may counteract the blood coagulation properties of vitamin K, increasing the risk of bleeding.

- **Reminder:** If you have a medical condition, talk to your doctor before taking supplements.

and reduce the blood level of LDL ("bad") cholesterol. But more research is needed to define the role of vitamin K in these and other disorders.

▼ HOW MUCH YOU NEED

An Adequate Intake (AI) has been established for vitamin K. Because vitamin K needs are met by the body, the daily AI is low: 120 mcg for men and 90 mcg for women age 19 and older.

IF YOU GET TOO LITTLE
In healthy people, a vitamin K deficiency is rare, because the body manufactures most of what it requires. In fact, deficiencies are found only in those with liver disease or intestinal illnesses that interfere with fat absorption. However, vitamin K levels can wane as a result of using antibiotics long term.

One of the first signs of a deficiency is a tendency to bruise easily. Those at risk need careful medical monitoring because they could bleed to death in the event of a serious injury.

IF YOU GET TOO MUCH
It's hard to get too much vitamin K because it's not abundant in any one food (except leafy greens). Although even megadoses are not toxic, high doses can be dangerous if you're taking anticoagulants. Large doses may also cause flushing and sweating.

▼ HOW TO TAKE IT

DOSAGE
Multivitamins often contain between 25 and 60 mcg of vitamin K. Bone-building formulas provide around 300 mcg a day, the equivalent of adding a large leafy salad to your daily diet. Higher doses (such as those in prenatal multivitamins) may be prescribed under medical supervision for those with specific medical needs.

GUIDELINES FOR USE
• When prescribed, vitamin K should be taken with meals. Food enhances its absorption.

▼ OTHER SOURCES

Leafy green vegetables, including—per cup of vegetable—kale (547 mcg), Swiss chard (299 mcg), and turnip greens (138 mcg), are richest in vitamin K. Broccoli, spring onions, and brussels sprouts are also good sources. Other foods with some vitamin K are pistachios, vegetable oils, meats, and dairy products.

FACTS & TIPS

■ If you take blood-thinning medications and eat lots of leafy green vegetables, which are rich in vitamin K, let your doctor know. The dose of your medication may need to be adjusted.

■ Vitamin E helps the body use vitamin K. But too much vitamin E—more than 1,000 IU a day—taken long term may impair vitamin K function and increase your risk of bleeding.

LATEST FINDINGS

■ Green tea is sometimes erroneously considered the leading source of vitamin K; it has 1,700 mcg in 8 ounces. Many doctors consequently advise their patients on anticoagulants (blood thinners) to skip the tea. In fact, that's the amount of vitamin K in 8 ounces of tea leaves—which would make hundreds of cups of brewed tea. According to a Tufts University study, a cup of green tea contains virtually no vitamin K.

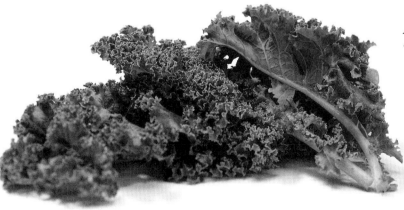

A cup of kale provides the equivalent of more than five 100 mcg tablets of vitamin K.

WHITE WILLOW BARK *(Salix alba)*

Used for thousands of years to treat fevers and headaches, white willow bark contains a chemical forerunner of today's most popular painkiller—aspirin. Effective for pain, inflammation, and fever, the herb is sometimes called "herbal aspirin," but fortunately causes few of that drug's side effects or complications.

COMMON USES

- Relieves acute and chronic pain.
- Reduces arthritis inflammation.
- May lower fevers.

FORMS

- Capsule
- Tablet
- Liquid
- Powder
- Dried herb/Tea

WHAT IT IS

White willow bark comes from the stately white willow tree, which can grow up to 75 feet tall. In China, its medicinal properties have been appreciated for centuries. But not until the eighteenth century was the herb recognized as a pain reliever and fever reducer in the West. European settlers brought the white willow tree to North America, where they discovered local tribes were using native willow species to alleviate pain and fight fevers.

In 1828 the plant's active ingredient, salicin, was isolated by German and French scientists, and 10 years later, European chemists manufactured salicylic acid, a chemical cousin to aspirin, from it. Regular aspirin, or acetylsalicylic acid, was later created from a different salicin-containing herb called meadowsweet.

By the end of the nineteenth century, the Bayer Company had begun commercially producing aspirin, which was marketed as a new and safer pain reliever than wintergreen and black birch oil, the herbs commonly employed at that time for reducing pain.

All parts of the white willow contain salicin, but concentrations of this chemical are highest in the bark, which is collected in early spring from trees that are two to five years old. *Salix alba*, or white willow, is the most popular species for medicinal use, but other types of willow are also rich in salicin, including *Salix fragilis* (crack willow), *Salix purpurea* (purple willow), and *Salix daphnoides* (violet willow). These species are often sold simply as willow bark in health-food stores.

▼ WHAT IT DOES

In the body, the salicin from white willow bark is metabolized to form salicylic acid, which reduces pain, fever, and inflammation. Though the herb is

▲ ALERT ▲

SIDE EFFECTS

- This herb rarely causes side effects at recommended doses.

- Higher doses can lead to an upset stomach, nausea, or tinnitus (ringing in the ears). If any of these reactions occur, lower the dosage or stop taking the herb. See your doctor if side effects persist.

CAUTION

- Do not consume white willow bark with aspirin because it can amplify the side effects of the drug. Additionally, anyone who has been told to avoid aspirin should also refrain from using white willow bark. This advice applies to people who are allergic to aspirin and to those with ulcers or other gastrointestinal disorders.

- Never give white willow bark to a child or teen under age 16 who has a cold, the flu, or chicken pox.

- Pregnant or breast-feeding women should consult their doctors before taking the herb; its safety has not been established in these situations.

- Avoid white willow bark if you also take an anticoagulant medication; there is an increased risk of bleeding.

- **Reminder:** If you have a medical condition, talk to your doctor before taking supplements.

slower acting than aspirin, its beneficial effects last longer, and it causes fewer adverse reactions. Most notably, it does not promote stomach bleeding—one of aspirin's potentially serious side effects.

MAJOR BENEFITS

White willow bark can be very effective for relieving headaches, as well as acute muscle aches and pains. It can also alleviate all sorts of chronic pain, including back and neck pain. When recommended for arthritis, especially if there is pain in the back, knees, and hips, it can reduce swelling and inflammation and increase joint mobility.

In addition, white willow bark may help ease the pain of menstrual cramps—the salicin interferes with the action of hormonelike chemicals called prostaglandins that can contribute to inflammation and cause pain.

ADDITIONAL BENEFITS

White willow bark, like aspirin, may be useful for bringing down fevers.

▼ HOW TO TAKE IT

DOSAGE

Take one or two pills three times a day, or as needed to relieve pain, lower a fever, or reduce inflammation (follow package instructions).

Look for preparations that are standardized to contain 15% salicin. This dosage provides between 60 and 120 mg a day of salicin. Standardized extracts can also be taken in liquid or powder form.

White willow bark teas are likely to be less effective than standardized extracts, because they supply only a small amount of pain-relieving salicin.

GUIDELINES FOR USE

• White willow bark is safe to use long term. It has a bitter, astringent taste, so the most convenient way to take it is probably in pill form.

• Taking aspirin puts youngsters with a fever at risk for a potentially fatal brain and liver condition called Reye's syndrome. Salicin, the therapeutic ingredient in white willow bark, is not likely to cause this problem because it is metabolized differently than aspirin. However, the herb's similarities to the painkiller warrant extra caution. For children and teens, acetaminophen is a better choice than white willow bark or aspirin.

SHOPPING HINTS

■ Buy white willow bark extract standardized to contain 15% salicin—the aspirinlike active ingredient in the herb.

■ Though white willow bark tea is sometimes recommended as a pain reliever, you should take only standardized extracts, in pill, powder, or liquid form. Because the bark contains 1% or less salicin, you'd probably have to drink at least several quarts of tea to get an effective dose.

■ If white willow bark doesn't help pain, try other pain-relieving herbs, such as meadowsweet, feverfew, cat's claw, or pau d'arco.

LATEST FINDINGS

■ A recent study confirms earlier reports that white willow bark appears to be quite safe. Among 41 patients with long-standing arthritis who were treated for two months with white willow bark (as well as other herbs), only three people taking the herbs had mild adverse reactions, including headache and digestive upset—all of which also occurred in those who were given a placebo.

DID YOU KNOW?

Native Americans and early settlers chewed willow twigs "until the ears ring" to relieve headache pain. Today, ringing in the ears is recognized as a sign that you've taken too much of the herb or its drug counterpart, aspirin.

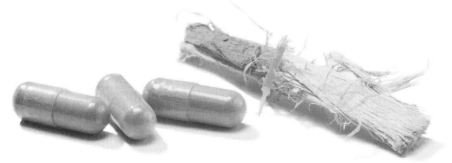

Bark from the white willow tree (dried, concentrated, and packaged into pills) is the source of a potent natural pain reliever.

ZINC

Everyone needs zinc. This mineral fuels enzymes that do everything from manufacturing DNA to healing wounds and keeping the body's hormones in balance. Zinc is a crucial component of a strong immune system, and it fights the common cold. Yet many Americans don't get enough of this vital nutrient.

COMMON USES

■ Fights colds, flu, other infections.

■ Treats a wide range of chronic ailments, from rheumatoid arthritis and underactive thyroid to fibromyalgia and osteoporosis.

■ Heals skin ailments and aids digestive complaints.

■ May boost fertility, build healthy hair, and diminish ringing in ears.

FORMS

■ Tablet

■ Capsule

■ Lozenge

■ Liquid

▼ WHAT IT IS

An essential mineral required by every cell in the body, zinc is concentrated in the muscles, bones, skin, kidneys, liver, pancreas, eyes, and in men, the prostate. It is plentiful in drinking water and in some foods, including meat. Because your body does not produce zinc, it depends on external sources for its supply.

▼ WHAT IT DOES

Zinc plays a critical role in hundreds of body processes—from cell growth and sexual maturation and immunity to the development of taste and smell. Consequently, everyone who takes a daily multivitamin and mineral supplement should be certain that it contains zinc. Individual supplements are also available for specific complaints.

MAJOR BENEFITS

Necessary for the proper functioning of the immune system, zinc helps to protect the body against colds, flu, conjunctivitis, and other infections. In a study of 100 people in the initial stages of a cold, those who sucked on zinc lozenges every couple of hours recovered from their illness about three days earlier than those who sucked on placebo lozenges. Zinc lozenges may also speed the healing of canker sores and sore throat.

Taken in pill form, zinc may aid in treating more serious illnesses, such as rheumatoid arthritis, lupus, fibromyalgia, and possibly multiple sclerosis, as well as other conditions, such as AIDS, which are associated with an improperly functioning immune system.

ADDITIONAL BENEFITS

Zinc exerts beneficial effects on various hormones, including the sex and thyroid hormones. It shows promise for enhancing fertility in both women and men. Zinc may also shrink an enlarged prostate. In addition, it may be effective for those with an underactive thyroid and, because it improves insulin levels, it may offer some benefits to people with diabetes.

Because zinc affects so many body systems, it has many other uses. It stimulates the healing of wounds and skin irritations, making it useful for acne, burns, eczema, psoriasis, and

ALERT

CAUTION

• Don't take too much zinc: More than 100 mg daily can, over the long term, impair immunity. It can also interfere with copper absorption, leading to anemia.

• Zinc supplements may alter the absorption and effectiveness of antibiotic drugs. Consult your doctor before taking them together.

• **Reminder:** If you have a medical condition, talk to your doctor before taking supplements.

rosacea, and promotes the health of the hair and scalp.

Zinc has also been shown to slow vision loss in people with macular degeneration, a common cause of blindness in those over age 50. And in a recent Japanese study, tinnitus (ringing in the ears) improved with zinc supplementation. Zinc may also be useful for osteoporosis, hemorrhoids, inflammatory bowel disease, and ulcers.

▼ HOW MUCH YOU NEED

The RDA for zinc is 8 mg for women and 11 mg for men daily. Higher doses are reserved for specific complaints.

IF YOU GET TOO LITTLE
Severe zinc deficiency is rare in the United States, but a mild zinc deficiency can lead to poor wound healing, more colds and flu, a muted sense of taste and smell, and skin problems such as acne, eczema, and psoriasis. It can result in impaired blood sugar tolerance (and an increased diabetes risk) and a low sperm count.

IF YOU GET TOO MUCH
Long-term use of more than 100 mg of zinc a day has been shown to impair immunity and lower levels of HDL ("good") cholesterol. One study reported a connection between excess zinc and Alzheimer's, though evidence is scant. Larger doses (more than

200 mg a day) can cause nausea, vomiting, and diarrhea.

▼ HOW TO TAKE IT

DOSAGE
The usual dosage is 30 mg once a day. Taking zinc for longer than a month may interfere with copper absorption, so add 2 mg of copper for every 30 mg of zinc.

For short-term use (colds or flu), use zinc lozenges every two to four hours for a week; don't exceed 150 mg a day.

GUIDELINES FOR USE
• Take zinc an hour before or two hours after a meal; if it causes stomach upset, have it with a low-fiber food.

• If you also use iron supplements, do not take them at the same time as zinc.

• Take zinc at least two hours after taking antibiotics.

▼ OTHER SOURCES

When looking for foods rich in zinc, think protein. It's abundant in beef, pork, liver, poultry (especially dark meat), eggs, and seafood (especially oysters). Cheese, beans, nuts, and wheat germ are other good sources, but the zinc in these foods is less easily absorbed than the zinc in meat.

SHOPPING HINTS
■ Zinc supplements come in many forms. When buying pills or liquids, zinc picolinate, acetate, citrate, glycerate, or monomethionine are all excellent choices; they're well absorbed and easy on the stomach. When shopping for lozenges to treat colds or flu, preparations containing zinc gluconate, ascorbate, or glycinate are your best bet.

LATEST FINDINGS
■ Zinc may be especially beneficial for older people who are often deficient in this mineral, according to a recent study of 118 elderly but relatively healthy nursing home residents in Rome, Italy. Those given 25 mg of zinc daily for three months showed improved immune systems. Experts think zinc may revitalize the thymus gland, which produces immune cells.

■ Studies show that exercisers lose zinc in perspiration and urine. That may be one reason why, although moderate exercise boosts immunity, long bouts of intense exercise are linked with lowered immunity.

DID YOU KNOW?
Almonds are a rich source of zinc for vegetarians, who may be deficient in it: 4 ounces provide about 6 mg–half the RDA of zinc for women.

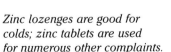

Zinc lozenges are good for colds; zinc tablets are used for numerous other complaints.

DRUG INTERACTIONS

Many people believe that herbs and other "natural" supplements are so gentle that they're safe to use under any circumstances. But in truth, a number of them interact in unwanted ways with prescription and over-the-counter (OTC) drugs, intensifying or blunting the action of the medications or even producing dangerous side effects.

Although research in the area of herb-drug interactions has increased, there is still much to be learned about the potential for problems.

To be safe, if you regularly take a prescription or OTC medication—or even another dietary supplement—consult your doctor before adding an herbal remedy to your regimen. After all, part of the reason that herbs can be so helpful is that they contain active (which can mean potentially interactive) ingredients.

In the same vein, if you have a medical or psychiatric condition, or are getting prepared for elective surgery, be sure to consult your doctor or pharmacist before trying any dietary supplement.

This section lists common drug classes and highlights interactions with popular dietary supplements that have been documented so far. While far from comprehensive, the list illustrates how real the risk for unwanted side effects and adverse reactions can be when combining drugs and herbs.

Even if you don't see the name of your particular drug listed, the interactions may still apply to all the drugs in that class. Always check the individual supplement profile in this book for specific information on any substance you are considering taking; current data on known interactions with common medications will be listed there.

ANTACIDS

The effectiveness and safety of **antacid medications** may be altered by the use of the following dietary supplements:
- **Iron** (take 2 hours before or after the antacid)
- **Vitamin D**

ANTIBIOTICS

A number of supplements may lessen the effectiveness of **oral antibiotics (doxycycline, minocycline, tetracycline,** and others). To reduce the risk of problems, take the supplement at least 2 hours before or after the antibiotic. Those supplements that may interact adversely with common oral antibiotics include:
- **Calcium**
- **Iron**
- **Magnesium**
- **Psyllium**
- **Zinc**

ANTICOAGULANTS

Certain supplements may interact dangerously with anticoagulants (blood-thinners) such as **warfarin** and daily **aspirin**, intensifying the effect of the medication and possibly leading to excessive bleeding. These supplements include:
- **Feverfew**
- **Fish oils**
- **Garlic**
- **Ginger**
- **Ginkgo biloba**
- **Reishi mushrooms**
- **Pau d'arco**
- **Vitamin E**
- **Vitamin K** (counteracts rather than intensifies the effects of the anticoagulant medication)
- **White willow bark**

ANTIDEPRESSANTS

There are a number of supplements that should not be taken with **antidepressants** of any type without consulting your doctor. Common medications in this category are **fluoxetine (Prozac), paroxetine (Paxil),** and **sertraline (Zoloft).** When these are used with the following supplements there is a risk of serious adverse interactions:
- **Melatonin**
- **St. John's wort**

Medications in the class of antidepressants known as **monoamine oxidase (MAO) inhibitors** such as **phenelzine (Nardil)** and **tranylcypromine (Parnate)** should not be taken within 14 days of certain dietary supplements due to a risk of anxiety, confusion, excessive sedation, and other potentially serious reactions. These supplements include:
- **Ephedra**
- **5-HTP**
- **Ginseng (Panax)**
- **St. John's wort**

ANTIHISTAMINES

Certain supplements may cause excessive drowsiness when taken with *sedating antihistamines.* These supplements include:

- **5-HTP**
- **Kava**
- **Melatonin**
- **Valerian**

CHOLESTEROL DRUGS

Cholesterol-lowering agents classified as *"statins" (lovastatin* and *simvastatin,* for example) should not be taken with certain supplements due to a risk of serious interactions. These supplements include:

- **Niacin**
- **Iron**
- **St. John's wort**

COLD REMEDIES

Prescription and over-the counter (OTC) remedies containing the drug *ephedrine* or *pseudoephedrine* should not be combined with the following supplements:

- **Ephedra**
- **5-HTP**

DIABETES DRUGS

Medications taken for diabetes, such as *insulin* and *oral diabetes drugs,* should be taken cautiously with certain supplements. There may be a risk of adverse side effects (such as enhanced blood sugar-lowering actions) and/or changes in the effectiveness of the medications. These supplements include:

- **Alpha-lipoic acid**
- **Cat's claw**
- **Chromium**
- **Dandelion**
- **Ephedra**
- **Ginseng (Panax)**
- **Siberian ginseng**

DIURETICS

Medications that reduce the amount of fluid in the body through increased urination are known as *diuretics.* There are three basic types: potassium-sparing, loop, and thiazide.

Agents classified as *potassium-sparing diuretics* (for example, the drugs *amiloride, spironolactone,* and *triamterene*) should not be taken with certain supplements without consulting your doctor due to a risk of hyperkalemia (too much potassium in the blood) and associated problems. These supplements include:

- **Phosphorus**
- **Potassium**

Agents classified as *loop diuretics* (for example, the drugs *bumetanide, ethacrynic acid, furosemide,* and *torsemide*) should not be used with certain supplements because of the risk of increasing or decreasing the drug's diuretic effect. These supplements include:

- **Dandelion**
- **Ephedra**
- **Ginseng (Panax)**
- **Glucosamine**

Agents classified as *thiazide diuretics* (for example, the drugs *clorothiazide, indapamide, hydrochlorothiazide,* and *metolazone*) should not be used with certain supplements because of the risk of increasing or decreasing the drug's diuretic effect, or in some cases causing serious side effects. These supplements include:

- **Aloe vera**
- **Calcium**
- **Dandelion**
- **Ephedra**
- **Glucosamine**
- **Hawthorn**
- **Licorice**
- **Potassium**

HEART AND BLOOD PRESSURE DRUGS

Many herbs and dietary supplements pose serious risks when taken together with prescription cardiac and antihypertensive (blood pressure-lowering) medications. Consult your doctor before combining any such medication with a dietary supplement. This precaution applies to any type of *calcium channel blocker, beta-blocker, ACE inhibitor, nitrate medication, digitalis drug,* or *cardiac glycoside (digitoxin* or *digoxin).* Notable and potentially serious interactions or side effects have been documented with the following supplements:

- **Aloe vera** (juice form)
- **Ephedra**
- **Garlic** (supplement form)
- **Ginseng (Panax** or **Siberian)**
- **Hawthorn**
- **Licorice**
- **Flavonoids** (specifically, a citrus bioflavonoid preparation containing naringin, a flavonoid present in grapefruit, but not in oranges)
- **Potassium**
- **Phosphorus**
- **St. John's wort**

MUSCLE RELAXANTS

Some supplements should not be combined with certain muscle relaxants (for example, the medications *carisoprodol, cyclobenzaprine,* and *metaxalone*) because there is a risk of causing excessive drowsiness, loss of alertness, and other unwanted reactions. These supplements include:

- **5-HTP**
- **Kava**
- **Melatonin**
- **Valerian**

NARCOTIC PAIN RELIEVERS

Certain supplements should not be taken with **codeine, hydrocodone/ acetaminophen,** or any other **narcotic analgesics** because excessive drowsiness and other dangerous complications may result. These supplements include:

- **5-HTP**
- **Goldenseal**
- **Kava**
- **Melatonin**
- **Valerian**

NEUROLOGY DRUGS

Risk of overstimulation, stomach upset, and other problems can occur when certain **nervous system stimulants,** such as **methylphenidate (Ritalin),** are combined with the following supplements:

- **Ephedra**
- **Ginseng (Panax)**

NSAIDS

Some supplements pose the risk of hyperkalemia (excessive amounts of potassium in the blood) if taken with **NSAIDs (nonsteroidal anti-inflammatory drugs)** such as **ibuprofen, ketoprofen,** and **naproxen,** for example. These supplements include:

- **Phosphorus**
- **Potassium**

Taken long-term, the NSAID **aspirin** carries the risk of excessive blood-thinning and bleeding when combined with certain supplements. These supplements include:

- **Feverfew**
- **Fish oils**
- **Garlic**
- **Ginkgo biloba**
- **Reishi mushrooms**
- **White willow bark**

OB/GYN DRUGS

Many supplements affect hormone levels and should be combined with **oral contraceptives**, **hormone replacement therapy medications**, and **other gynecological drugs** only after discussion with a doctor. Interactions could lessen the potency of the drug or even cause harm. These supplements include:

- **Black cohosh**
- **Cat's claw**
- **Chasteberry**
- **Soy isoflavones**
- **St. John's wort**

PARKINSON'S DRUGS

Two supplements in particular pose a risk of interactions when taken with the anti-Parkinson medication **levodopa**. Consult your doctor before combining. These supplements are:

- **5-HTP**
- **Vitamin B$_6$**

PSYCHIATRIC DRUGS

Certain supplements can interfere with the action of a wide range of psychiatric medications such as **antipsychotic, antianxiety,** and **antimanic drugs.** These supplements include:

- **Ginseng (Panax)**
- **Iodine**
- **Kava**
- **5-HTP**

SEDATIVES/TRANQUILIZERS

Excessive drowsiness and other side effects associated with alertness and concentration have occurred when **sleep aids** and other **sedatives** and **tranquilizers** have been taken with the following supplements:

- **Black cohosh**
- **5-HTP**
- **Goldenseal**
- **Kava**
- **Melatonin**
- **Valerian**

SEIZURE/EPILEPSY DRUGS

The effect of some anticonvulsants (for example, the drugs **phenytoin, carbamazepine,** and **gabapentin**) may be compromised if you are using the following B-vitamin supplements:

- **Folic acid**
- **Vitamin B$_6$**

Corticosteroids taken orally (for example, the drugs **beclomethasone** and **prednisone**) should not be combined with certain supplements because of the risk of adverse interactions. These supplements include:

- **Aloe vera** (juice form)
- **Ginseng (Panax)**
- **Melatonin**
- **Phosphorus**

THYROID DRUGS

Common thyroid medications (for example, the drugs **methimazole** and **propylthiouracil**) should not be used with certain supplements because of the risk of adverse interactions or reduced effectiveness of the prescription medication. These supplements include:

- **Iodine**
- **Kelp**

Acute Short, severe, nonchronic; designates an illness or condition that typically lasts no more than a week or two.

Alternative medicine Any of various approaches to healing, such as herbal therapies and acupuncture, that fall outside the domain of conventional mainstream medicine.

Amino acids Chemical substances, found in foods and produced in the body, which are used to build protein.

Antibiotic A drug that kills or inhibits infection-causing bacteria.

Anticoagulant A drug (such as warfarin or daily aspirin) that deters blood clotting; often used by those at risk for heart attacks. Also known as a blood thinner.

Anticonvulsant A drug that prevents seizures; used to treat epilepsy.

Anti-inflammatory A drug or supplement that fights inflammation, which is a response to injury or irritation that is characterized by redness, heat, swelling, and pain.

Antioxidant A substance that protects cells from the damaging effects of highly reactive oxygen molecules called free radicals. Some antioxidants, such as alpha-lipoic acid, are made by the body; others, such as vitamins C and E, are obtained through diet or supplements.

Antispasmodic A drug or supplement that prevents spasms or cramps in the digestive tract or elsewhere.

Beta-blocker A type of drug that affects the heart, blood vessels, and other areas; often prescribed to treat high blood pressure or angina.

Botanical An herb or plant that has healing properties.

Botanical name The scientific, or Latin, name of an herb or plant.

Chronic Persistent or long term; designates an illness or condition that often requires months or years of treatment for results to be apparent.

Coenzyme A substance that acts in concert with enzymes to speed up chemical reactions in the body.

Commission E A special body of scientists, health professionals, and lay experts formed in Germany in 1978; it studies the usefulness and safety of herbal remedies.

Complex A term designating a mixture of vitamins, minerals, herbs, or other nutrients. Examples include vitamin B complex, liver (lipotropic) complex, and amino acid complex.

Compress A soft cotton or flannel cloth or piece of gauze soaked in an herbal tea or other healing substance, then folded and placed on the skin to help reduce inflammation and pain.

Conventional medicine Also known as allopathic medicine, the approach to healing most commonly practiced in the United States and other Western countries. A doctor diagnoses a problem and typically treats it with drugs and/or surgery.

Douche Herbal teas, acidophilus and water, or other substances that can be used to flush the vagina; may be recommended for infections.

Endorphins Natural pain-reducing substances released by the pituitary gland, producing an effect similar to that of narcotic pain relievers.

Enteric coating A protective covering that enables a pill to pass intact through the stomach into the small intestine, where the coating dissolves and the contents are best absorbed.

Enzyme A protein that speeds up specific chemical reactions and processes in the body, such as digestion and energy production.

Essential Fatty Acids (EFAs) The building blocks that the body uses to make fats. The body must get various kinds of EFAs through diet or supplements (such as fish oils and flaxseed oil) to assure proper health.

Essential oil A concentrated oil extracted from herbs or other plants.

Extract A pill, powder, liquid, or other form of an herb that contains a concentrated, and usually standard, amount of therapeutic ingredients.

Food and Drug Administration (FDA) The United States government agency that regulates and monitors the safety of foods and drugs (but not dietary supplements).

Free radicals Highly reactive and unstable oxygen molecules, generated in the body, that can damage cells, leading to heart disease, cancer, and other ailments. Antioxidants help minimize free-radical damage.

Gram A metric measure of weight, sometimes used in dosages. There are 1,000 milligrams (mg) in 1 gram, and 28.35 grams in an ounce.

Herb A plant or plant part—the leaves, stems, roots, bark, or flowers—that can be used for medicinal or other purposes (such as flavoring foods).

Hormone Any of various chemical messengers, produced by the adrenal, pituitary, thyroid, ovaries, testes, and other glands, that have far-reaching effects throughout the body. Hormones regulate everything from growth and tissue repair to metabolism, reproduction, blood pressure, and the body's response to stress.

Integrative medicine An approach to healing that utilizes aspects of both conventional and alternative medicine. Also called complementary medicine.

International Unit (IU) A standardized dose measure that provides a set amount of a specific supplement, such as vitamin A, D, or E.

Lipotropic combination A blend of choline, inositol, methionine, milk thistle, and other nutrients used to promote the health of the liver.

Metabolism The cascading array of chemical reactions by which the body converts food into packets of energy that can be used or stored.

Microgram (mcg) A metric measure of weight used in dosages. There are 1,000 mcg in 1 milligram (mg).

Milligram (mg) A metric measure of weight used in dosages. There are 1,000 mg in 1 gram.

Mineral An inorganic substance found in the earth's crust that plays a crucial role in the human body for enzyme creation, regulation of heart rhythm, bone formation, and other processes.

Mixed amino acids A balanced blend (complex) of amino acids, often taken in conjunction with individual amino acid supplements.

Monoamine Oxidase (MAO) Inhibitor A specific class of drugs used to treat depression. MAO inhibitors frequently interact with various foods, drugs, and dietary supplements.

Mucilage A gummy, gel-like plant substance that when ingested forms a protective layer in the throat and digestive tract, suppressing coughs and adding bulk to hard stools.

Neurotransmitter Any of various chemicals found in the brain and throughout the body that transmit signals among nerve cells.

Nonsteroidal Anti-inflammatory Drug (NSAID) A drug—such as aspirin, ibuprofen, or naproxen—that reduces pain and inflammation by blocking the production of prostaglandins (see also Prostaglandins).

Nutritional supplement A nutrient, synthesized in the lab or extracted from plants or animals and taken for medicinal purposes.

PCOs (Procyanidolic Oligomers) A group of antioxidant compounds, also called proanthocyanidins—found in pine bark, grape seed extract, green tea, red wine, and other substances—that may help protect against heart and vascular disease.

Phytoestrogens Estrogenlike compounds present in soy and other plants that may help treat symptoms of menopause, certain cancers, and other complaints.

Phytomedicines Therapeutic ingredients found in fruits, vegetables, grains, herbs, and other plants that may help protect against cancer, heart disease, and other ailments.

Placebo Also called a dummy pill, a substance that contains no medicinal ingredients. Often used in scientific studies as a control so its effects can be compared with those of the drug or supplement under scrutiny.

Poultice A soft, moist substance, spread between layers of cloth or gauze, that is applied (usually heated) to the skin in order to help reduce pain and inflammation.

Probiotics "Friendly" bacteria, similar to those found in acidophilus supplements, that are normally present in the intestine and help to promote healthy digestion.

Prolactin A hormone secreted by the pituitary gland in the brain that promotes lactation.

Prostaglandins Hormonelike chemicals occurring naturally in the body and producing a wide range of effects, such as inducing inflammation, stimulating uterine contractions during labor, and protecting the lining of the stomach.

Recommended Dietary Allowance (RDA) The daily amount of a vitamin or mineral needed by healthy individuals to meet the body's needs and prevent a deficiency. These guidelines are set by the Food and Nutrition Board of the National Academy of Sciences.

Standardized extract A concentrated form of an herb that contains a set (standardized) level of active ingredients. Standardization helps guarantee a consistent dosage strength, or potency, from one batch of herb to the next. Standardized extracts are available only for certain herbs, either as pills or liquids or in other forms.

Sublingual Beneath the tongue. Some supplements, such as vitamin B_{12}, are formulated to dissolve in the mouth, providing quick absorption into the bloodstream without interference from stomach acids.

Therapeutic dose The amount of a vitamin, mineral, herb, nutritional supplement, or drug needed to produce a desired healing effect (as opposed to the minimum amount needed to prevent a deficiency—such as the RDA, for example).

Tonic An herb (such as ginseng) or herbal blend that is used to "tone" the body or a specific organ, imparting added strength or vitality.

Vitamin An organic substance that plays an essential role in regulating cell functions in the body. Most vitamins must be ingested, because the body cannot produce them.

INDEX

▼